THIRD EDITION
CASE REVIEWS IN
OPHTHALMOLOGY

Neil J. Friedman, MD
Adjunct Clinical Professor
Department of Ophthalmology, Stanford University School of Medicine
Palo Alto, CA, USA
Partner, Mid-Peninsula Ophthalmology Medical Group
Menlo Park, CA, USA

Peter K. Kaiser, MD
Chaney Family Endowed Chair for Ophthalmology Research
Professor of Ophthalmology
Cleveland Clinic Lerner College of Medicine
Cole Eye Institute, Cleveland Clinic,
Cleveland, OH, USA

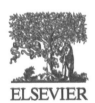

ELSEVIER

Elsevier
1600 John F. Kennedy Blvd.
Ste 1800
Philadelphia, PA 19103-2899

CASE REVIEWS IN OPHTHALMOLOGY, THIRD EDITION ISBN: 978-0-323-79409-1

Notice

Practitioners and researchers must always rely on their own experience and knowledge in evaluating and using any information, methods, compounds or experiments described herein. Because of rapid advances in the medical sciences, in particular, independent verification of diagnoses and drug dosages should be made. To the fullest extent of the law, no responsibility is assumed by Elsevier, authors, editors or contributors for any injury and/or damage to persons or property as a matter of products liability, negligence or otherwise, or from any use or operation of any methods, products, instructions, or ideas contained in the material herein.

Previous editions copyrighted 2012, and 2018.

Senior Content Strategist: Kayla Wolfe
Senior Content Development Specialist: Shweta Pant
Publishing Services Manager: Deepthi Unni
Senior Project Manager: Manchu Mohan
Book Designer: Ryan Cook

Printed in the United States of America.

Last digit is the print number: 9 8 7 6 5 4 3 2

Working together
to grow libraries in
developing countries

www.elsevier.com • www.bookaid.org

CASE REVIEWS IN
OPHTHALMOLOGY

Preface

The third edition of *Case Reviews in Ophthalmology* builds on the foundation we originally created: a case-based approach to ophthalmic topics. We updated the book by presenting new cases in every section, revising existing cases to reflect the latest treatment and management guidelines, and including additional figures to enhance the previous material. We believe this new text will improve your study experience and provide a more comprehensive educational aid for the vast quantity of information that we are required to master.

We hope that these cases continue to be helpful for understanding clinical problems and preparing for exams.

Neil J. Friedman, MD
Peter K. Kaiser, MD

Acknowledgments

We are grateful to our colleagues, friends, and family who helped in the preparation of this new edition.

We are fortunate to work with a first-rate publishing group at Elsevier: thank you Kayla Wolfe, Nani Clansey, Laura Klein, Shweta Pant, Manchu Mohan, and your wonderful team.

And of course, we are most thankful to our families: Mae, Jake, Dawn, Peter (PJ), and Stephanie for their encouragement, love, and support.

Neil J. Friedman, MD
Peter K. Kaiser, MD

Contents

Abbreviations

A

ABMD – anterior basement membrane dystrophy
ACD – anterior chamber depth
ACE – angiotensin-converting enzyme
ACh – acetylcholine
AD – autosomal dominant
AION – anterior ischemic optic neuropathy
AKC – atopic keratoconjunctivitis
AL – axial length
ALK – anterior lamellar keratoplasty
AMD – age-related macular degeneration
ANA – anti-nuclear antibody
ANCA – anti-neutrophil cytoplasmic antibody
APMPPE – acute posterior multifocal placoid pigment epitheliopathy
AR – autosomal recessive
A-ROP – aggressive ROP
AREDS – Age-Related Eye Disease Study
ARMD – age-related macular degenerations
ARN – acute retinal necrosis
AV – arteriovenous
AVM – arteriovenous malformation

B

BAT – brightness acuity
BCC – basal cell carcinoma
BCVA – best-corrected visual acuity
BO – baseout
BP – blood pressure
BRVO – Branch retinal vein occlusion
BSCVA – best spectacle-corrected visual acuity
BUN – blood urea nitrogen
BVOS – Branch Vein Occlusion Study

C

CAI – carbonic anhydrase inhibitor
CBC – complete blood count
CHED – congenital hereditary endothelial dystrophy
CHRPE – congenital hypertrophy of the RPE
CHSD – congenital hereditary stromal dystrophy
CIN – conjunctivital intraepithelial neoplasia
CK – conducive keratoplasty

CME – cystoid macular edema
CMV – cytomegalovirus
CN – cranial nerve
CNS – central nervous system
CNV – choroidal neovascularization
CNTGS – Collaborative Normal Tension Glaucoma Study
CPEO – chronic progressive external ophthalmoplegia
CRP – C-reactive protein
CRVO – central retinal vein occlusion
CSC – central serous chorioretinopathy
CSME – clinically significant macular edema
CT – computed tomography
CTA – computed tomography angiography
CVK – computerized videokeratography
CVOS – Central Vein Occlusion Study
CWS – cotton-wool spot
CXL – corneal collagen cross-linking

D

DALK – deep ALK
DCCT – Diabetes Control and Complications Trial
DED – dry eye disease
DLK – diffuse lamellar keratitis
DMAEK – Descemet membrane automated endothelial keratoplasty
DME – diabetic macular edema
DMEK – Descemet Membrane Endothelial Keratoplasty
DRCR.net – Diabetic Retinopathy Clinical Research Network
DRS – Diabetic Retinopathy Study
DSAEK – Descemet Stripping Automated Endothelial Keratoplasty
DSEK – Descemet Stripping Endothelial Keratoplasty
DUSN – diffuse unilateral subacute neuroretinitis
DVD – dissociated vertical deviation

E

EBMD – epithelial basement membrane dystrophy
EBV – Epstein–Barr virus
ECCE – extracapsular cataract extraction
EDOF – extended depth of focus
EDTA – ethylene diamine tetra-acetic acid

EK – endothelial keratoplasty
EKC – epidemic keratoconjunctivitis
ELISA – enzyme-linked immunosorbent assay
ELP – effective lens position
EMG – electromyography
EOG – electrooculogram
EOM – extraocular muscle
ER – emergency room
ERG - electroretinogram
ERM – epiretinal membrane
ESR – erythrocyte sedimentation rate
ET – esotropia
ETDRS – Early Treatment Diabetic Retinopathy Study
ETROP – Early Treatment of ROP
EVS – Endophthalmitis Vitrectomy Study

F

FA – fluorescein angiogram
FAF – fundus autofluorescence
FEVR – familial exudative vitreoretinopathy
FBS – foreign body sensation
FTA-ABS – fluorescent treponemal antibody absorption
FTMH – full-thickness macular hole

G

GA – geographic atrophy
GCA – giant cell arteritis
GPC – giant papillary conjunctivitis

H

HEDS – Herpetic Eye Disease Study
HIV – human immunodeficiency virus
HSV – herpes simplex virus
HVF – Humphrey visual field
HZO – herpes zoster ophthalmicus

I

ICCE – intracapsular cataract extraction
ICE – iridocorneal endothelial
ICG – indocyanine green
IFA – indirect immunofluorescence assay
IFIS – intraoperative floppy iris syndrome
IIH – idiopathic intracranial hypertension
IK – interstitial keratitis
INO – internuclear ophthalmoplegia
IOFD – intraocular foreign body
IOI – idiopathic orbital inflammation
IOL – intraocular lens
IOP – intraocular pressure

IPD – interpupillary distance
IRMA – intraretinal microvascular abnormality
IV - intravenous

K

KC – keratoconus
KP – keratic precipitates

L

LASIK – laser-assisted in situ keratomileusis
LHON – Leber hereditary optic neuropathy
LP – light perception or light projection
LP – lumbar puncture
LTK – laser thermal keratoplasty

M

MALT – mucosa-associated lymphoma tissue
MCP – multifocal choroiditis and panuveitis
MDF – map-dot-fingerprint
MEWDS – multiple evanescent white dot syndrome
mfERG – multifocal ERG
MG – myasthenia gravis
MGD – Meibomian gland dysfunction
MHA-TP – microhemagglutination assay for *Treponema
pallidum*
MLF – medial longitudinal fasciculus
MMP – matrix metalloproteinase
MRA – magnetic resonance angiography
MRD – margin reflex distance
MRI – magnetic resonance imaging
MS – multiple sclerosis
MUTT – Mycotic Ulcer Treatment Trial

N

NAION – non-arteritic anterior ischemic optic neuropathy
NF - neurofibromatosis
NFL – nerve fiber layer
NICU – neonatal intensive care unit
NLDO – nasolacrimal duct obstruction
NPDR – nonproliferative diabetic retinopathy
NSAID – nonsteroidal anti-inflammatory drug
NTG – normal tension glaucoma
NVD – neovascularization of the disc
NVG – neovascular glaucoma

O

OCP – ocular cicatricial pemphigoid
OCT – optical coherence tomography
OCTA – OCT angiography
OD – right eye

OKN – optokinetic nystagmus
ON – optic nerve
ONTT – Optic Neuritis Treatment Trial
OS – left eye
OU – both eyes
OVD – ophthalmic viscosurgical device

P

PAM – potential acuity meter
PAM – primary acquired melanosis
PAS – peripheral anterior synechiae
PBK – pseudophakic bullous keratopathy
PCO – posterior capsular opacity
PCR – polymerase chain reaction
PCV – polypoidal choroidal vasculopathy
PD – prism diopter
PDR – proliferative diabetic retinopathy
PDS – pigment dispersion syndrome
PDS – port delivery system
PDT – photodynamic therapy
PERK – prospective evaluation of radial keratotomy
PG – pigmentary glaucoma
PHN – postherpetic neuralgia
PHPV – persistent hyperplastic primary vitreous
PIC – punctuate inner choroiditis
PIOL – primary intraocular lymphoma
PK – penetrating keratoplasty
PMR – polymyalgia rheumatica
POAG – primary open-angle glaucoma
POHS – presumed ocular histoplasmosis syndrome
PORN – progressive outer retinal necrosis
PPCD – posterior polymorphous corneal dystrophy
PPD – purified protein derivative
PPRF – paramedian pontine reticular formation
PRK – photoreactive keratectomy
PRP – pan-retinal photocoagulation
PSC – posterior subcapsular cataract
PTK – phototherapeutic keratectomy
PTT – partial thromboplastin time
PVD – posterior vitreous detachment
PVRL – primary vitreoretinal lymphoma
PXG – pseudoexfoliative glaucoma
PXS – pseudoexfoliation syndrome

R

RAPD – relative afferent pupillary defect
RB – retinoblastoma
RD – retinal detachment
RF – rheumatoid factor

RGP – rigid gas permeable
RLE – refractive lens exchange
ROP – retinopathy of prematurity
RPE – retinal pigment epithelium
RPR – rapid plasma reagin
RRD – rhegmatogenous retinal detachment
RVO – retinal vein occlusion

S

SALK – superficial ALK
SCL – soft contact lens
SEI – subepithelial infiltrate
SJS – Stevens–Johnson syndrome
SLE – systemic lupus erythematosus
SMILE – small incision lenticule extraction
SO – superior oblique
SPEP – serum protein electrophoresis
SRF – subretinal fluid
STD – sexually transmitted disease

T

TASS – toxic anterior segment syndrome
TED – thyroid eye disease
TSH – thyroid-stimulating hormone
TRD – traction retinal detachment
TRIC – trachoma-inclusion conjunctivitis
TSI – thyroid-stimulating immunoglobulin

U

UBM – ultrasound biomicroscopy
UKPDS – United Kingdom Prospective Diabetes Study
URI – upper respiratory infection

V

VDRL – Venereal Disease Research Laboratory
VEGF – vascular endothelial growth factor
VEP – visual evoked potential
VER – visual evoked response
VF – visual field
VKC – vernal keratoconjunctivitis
VKH – Vogt–Koyanagi–Harada
VMA – vitreomacular adhesion
VMT – vitreomacular traction
VMTS – vitreomacular traction syndrome
VZV – varicella zoster virus

X

XT - exotropia

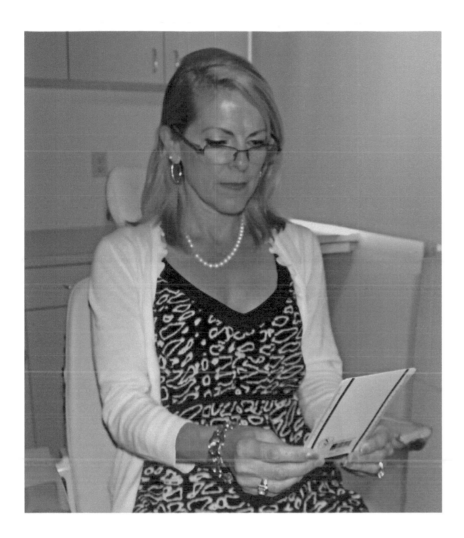

A 48-year-old woman with myopia complains of progressive deterioration in distance and near vision in both eyes for the past 2 years. She can improve her vision by sliding her glasses down her nose. Her past medical history is significant for diabetes for 10 years, for which she takes glyburide. She reports blood sugar levels usually between 120 and 140 mg/dL and a recent hemoglobin A1c of 6.8%.

1. What is the differential diagnosis?
2. What other history would you like to know?
3. What would your exam entail?

Additional information: her current glasses are –5.00 D with an add of +1.25 D OU, her manifest refraction is –4.25 D OD and –4.50 D OS with +1.50 D add OU. The crystalline lenses are clear OU and there is no diabetic retinopathy. Cycloplegic refraction reveals –4.25 D OU.

4. What is your diagnosis and treatment plan?

1. Decreased myopia and increased presbyopia. The change in refractive error may be due to overcorrection in her current distance spectacle prescription, cataracts, diabetic macular edema, or medications (ie, chloroquine, phenothiazines, antihistamines, benzodiazepines).

2. How old is her current prescription and what type of glasses are they? Does she have glare/halo/starburst from lights? Has the diabetes ever affected her retina and if so did she ever have any retinal treatment? Is she taking any other medications?

3. Measure her current glass prescription, perform a manifest refraction, and then a complete eye exam with attention to the crystalline lens for cataract and retina for diabetic macular edema.

4. Myopia/presbyopia with overminused glasses. A new glasses prescription should be given using the power from her manifest refraction. She should continue good blood sugar control and return for annual eye exams.

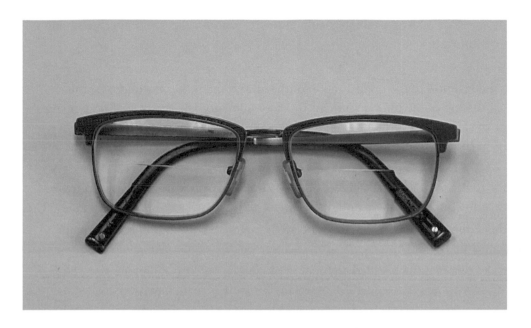

A 50-year-old man notices more difficulty reading and working on the computer. He uses his wife's "cheaters," which help.

1. What are his spectacle options?
2. What are the two prismatic effects that occur with bifocals?
3. Discuss the advantages and disadvantages of different bifocal designs.
4. What are the alternatives to glasses for correcting presbyopia?

1. The glasses options are progressive, bifocal, or single vision lenses. Glasses for the computer can be single vision, trifocal, or computer bifocals.

2. Image jump and image displacement.

   Image jump is related to the position of the optical center of the add segment. It is produced by the sudden prismatic power at the top of the bifocal segment (it is not influenced by the type of underlying lens). As the patient's line of sight crosses from the optical center of the distance lens to the bifocal segment, the image position suddenly shifts up owing to the base-down prismatic effect of the bifocal segment.

   Image displacement is due to the total prismatic power of the lens and bifocal segment. It is minimized when the prismatic effect of the bifocal segment and distance lens are in opposite directions.

   Image jump is more bothersome than image displacement, so the segment type should be chosen to minimize image jump.

3. The advantage of progressive lenses is the blended segment without a visible line and there is no image jump; however, there is usually an adaptation period, especially for patients who have previously worn lined bifocals.

   Bifocal lenses have a visible line and there are different types of segment styles – round-top, flat-top, and executive. Round-top segments produce the most image jump, and they cause more image displacement in myopes than in hyperopes. Flat-top segments minimize image jump, and image displacement is less in a myope than in a hyperope. Executive bifocals have a larger area dedicated to near vision, and there is no image jump because the optical centers are at the top of the segment.

4. *Contact lenses*: monovision or bifocal/multifocal lenses.

   Medication: topical miotic eyedrops to constrict pupil and increase depth of field.

   Surgery: laser vision correction (monovision or presbyopic ablation [outside United States], corneal inlay (nondominant eye), scleral procedure (incisions, laser, implants), RLE monovision or bifocal/multifocal/accommodating IOL.

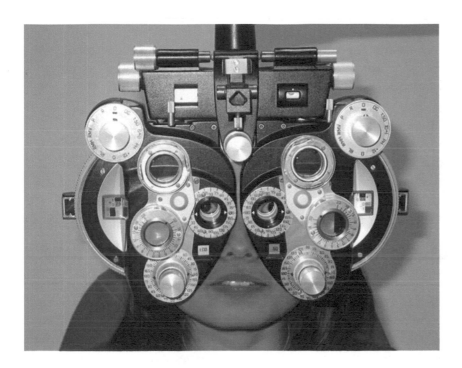

A 46-year-old woman complains of trouble with near vision. Her current glasses are 4 years old and she says her eyes feel strained when she reads. She wants to get a new prescription for glasses.

1. What is the technique for subjective manifest refraction?
2. How would you determine her add power?

1. Starting with her current prescription in either a trial lens or phoropter, the distance vision is checked monocularly and the sphere is adjusted first as she is asked to read progressively smaller lines on the acuity chart. The axis of any cylinder is then refined with a Jackson cross cylinder. The vision must be at least 20/40 to use the 0.25 cross cylinder. Once the correct axis is determined, the amount of cylinder is then determined in a similar fashion with the cross cylinder. The sphere is then rechecked until the best acuity is achieved. Finally, three methods can be used to perform binocular balance to equally control accommodation in both eyes during distance refraction: prism dissociation (3 PD base-up over one eye and 3 PD base-down over the other with a Risley prism), balanced fogging (fog both eyes and alternate cover until equally fogged), or duochrome test (red–green balance both eyes).

2. To determine the bifocal add, measure accommodation monocularly then binocularly. A Prince rule (reading card with a ruler calibrated in centimeters and diopters to measure amplitude of accommodation) can be used with the phoropter to determine the necessary accommodative requirement for various near vision tasks. Half of the patient's measured accommodative amplitude should be held in reserve to prevent asthenopia.

   For example, if the patient desires to read at 40 cm (2.5 D), the Prince rule measures 2.0 D of amplitude (1.0 D is available to patient to prevent asthenopic symptoms), then the add power is 1.5 D (the difference between accommodation [1.0 D] and the total amount of accommodation required to read [2.5 D]). With the calculated add in front of the distance correction, measure the accommodative range (near point to far point of accommodation). If the range is too close, then reduce the add in steps of 0.25 D until the correct range is found.

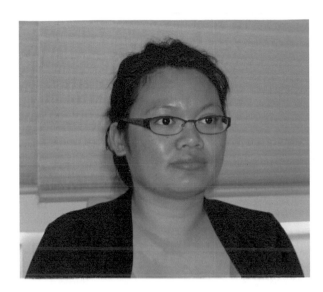

A 31-year-old woman with a refractive error of –2.50 D in both eyes is interested in refractive surgery. She has become contact lens intolerant and glasses interfere with her sports activities and lifestyle.

1. What would you tell her about surgical correction of her myopia?
2. What are the complications of LASIK?

Additional information: this patient undergoes LASIK. The day after surgery, she is very happy with her 20/20 vision. On exam, her left eye has the finding seen in the photo.

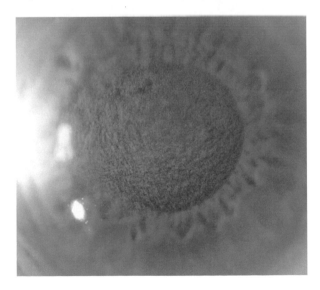

3. What is the diagnosis and how is it classified?
4. How would you treat this?

1. There are a number of surgical options for correcting low myopia. The most common is excisional (laser vision correction [surface ablation, LASIK, SMILE]). Other techniques include incisional (RK) and additive (implants [Intacs]). The indications, risks, benefits, alternatives, and complications of surgery should be discussed as well as the advantages and disadvantages of each of the procedures. She should also be told about what to expect during the preoperative and postoperative periods.

2. LASIK complications include: over- or undercorrection, glare/halos at night, dry eye, irregular/poor flap (too thick or thin, button-hole, incomplete, free cap), epithelial defect, decentered ablation, irregular astigmatism, flap dislocation, striae, epithelial ingrowth, interface inflammation (DLK), central toxic keratopathy, infection, scarring, and keratectasia. Late DLK may occur (any time in the future) after a corneal abrasion.

3. DLK, stage 2. Classification is as follows:

   Stage 1: peripheral inflammatory cells (usually postop day 1–2).

   Stage 2: inflammatory cells migrate centrally (usually postop day 3–4).

   Stage 3: more central inflammatory cells with scarring.

   Stage 4: stomal melting and scarring.

4. Frequent topical steroids. Steroid eye drops should be prescribed initially every hour while awake and steroid ointment at bedtime. The eye should be checked daily for improvement, and the steroids are tapered as the DLK resolves. If the interface inflammation progresses to stage 3 or 4, then the flap should be lifted and the stromal bed irrigated. A short course of oral steroids may also be given.

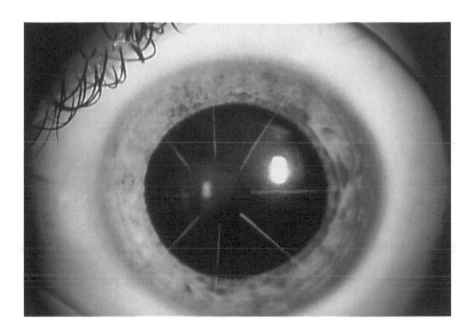

A 50-year-old man reports a history of RK surgery 20 years ago. He has noted glare and starbursts at night since the surgery. He used to experience fluctuating vision but says this has improved. He also notes that his vision has gradually deteriorated, especially over the last 10 years, and he needs stronger glasses for better reading as well as distance vision.

1. What would you specifically look for on exam?
2. What would you tell him about his symptoms?
3. What are the treatment options?

1. Manifest refraction, pupil size in dim and bright light, the corneal status (number of RK incisions and optical zone size, central irregularity, scarring, dryness), presence of cataract, and macular pathology. If there is visual fluctuation throughout the day, then morning and afternoon refractions should be performed.

2. Glare/starbursts are common after RK, particularly with smaller optical zones. The deep radial corneal incisions change the shape of the cornea but also weaken the cornea and can produce fluctuations in vision throughout the day and from day to day as refractive shifts occur. Altitude and humidity changes can exacerbate the fluctuations. Over time, many RK patients develop a progressive hyperopic shift (PERK study 10-year results found 43% of patients had at least a 1 D shift). In addition, this patient is presbyopic and is noting the combined effect of progressive hyperopia from the RK plus increasing presbyopia.

3. Treatment options include correction of any refractive error and pharmacologic (alphagan or pilocarpine) to reduce pupil size and decrease nighttime glare/starburst. He may need different glasses for different times of the day depending on the amount of fluctuation. If the refractive error is stable, then surface ablation can be performed with topical mitomycin C (to prevent scarring). If his symptoms are due to a cataract, then cataract surgery should be discussed and the patient informed that the refractive outcome is less predictable because of his previous RK surgery (eg, accurately measuring central corneal power), and therefore he may require a second procedure (laser vision correction, piggyback IOL, or IOL exchange) to correct a significant residual refractive error.

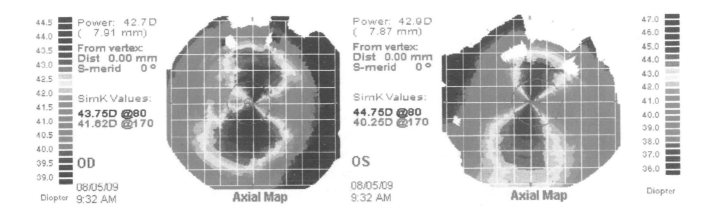

A patient with astigmatism complains of problems adapting to her new glasses and says she can see better with her old glasses. Her old prescription is −5.00 +2.00 × 85 OD and −6.50 +3.50 × 85 OS; her new prescription is −5.25 +2.25 × 95 OD and −7.50 +4.25 × 80 OS.

1. How would you address her complaint?

2. What does the corneal topography show?

3. What is the typical natural history of corneal astigmatism?

4. How is astigmatism corrected surgically?

1. The new glasses should be measured with a lensometer to confirm that the prescription is correct, the ocular alignment of the lenses checked, and the visual acuity recorded. The manifest refraction should then be rechecked carefully, and consider performing a cycloplegic refraction. If there is an error in the glasses or lens alignment, then simply remaking the lenses may resolve the problem. If the repeat manifest or cycloplegic refraction is different from the glasses prescription, then a new prescription should be given to the patient. Finally, patients with large levels of correction are particularly sensitive to small changes in their glasses prescription (ie, >0.50 D and/or >5 degrees axis rotation), and the vertex distance and base curve of the lenses must also be taken into account. Therefore, it may be necessary to make only a small change in the prescription at a time until the full change can be tolerated. When there is a significant change in the prescription, the patient should be told of this and warned that it may take some time to adapt to the new glasses.

2. The corneal topography demonstrates regular with-the-rule astigmatism, which appears as a vertically oriented symmetric bowtie. According to the SimK values, there is 2.13 D of astigmatism in the 80 degree meridian OD and 4.50 D of astigmatism in the 80 degree meridian OS.

3. Corneal astigmatism tends to be with-the-rule in children and typically decreases with age. Adults tend to have against-the-rule astigmatism that increases with age. Approximately 50% of the population has 0.75 D or more of astigmatism. The total astigmatism in the eye is the sum of that in the cornea (anterior and posterior surfaces [posterior contributes approximately 0.4 D against-the-rule]), the lens, and rarely the retina.

4. *Keratorefractive*: incisions (astigmatic keratotomy, corneal/limbal relaxing incisions) with a blade or laser, ablation (PRK, LASIK), and lenticule extraction (SMILE).

   Lenticular: toric IOL (phakic IOL or pseudophakic IOL).

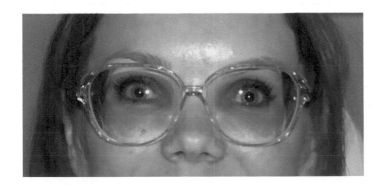

A 38-year-old myopic woman complains that her bulky, heavy glasses are a nuisance and she would like to investigate other options.

1. What are the alternatives and what other information would you like to know?

Additional information: she has worn glasses for 30 years, the last change was 7 years ago, she is not interested in contact lenses, has no other eye problems, and has not noticed a recent change in vision. Her current glasses are −7.25 +1.00 × 100 OD and −8.00 +2.50 × 20 OS, her vision with these glasses is 20/20 OU, her refraction yields the same prescription and vision. There is no evident anterior or posterior segment abnormality on slit-lamp exam and ophthalmoscopy. She is interested in refractive surgery.

2. What surgical options are available and what tests would you perform?

Additional information: corneal pachymetry is thinnest centrally and measures 505 μm OD and 510 μm OS, angles are open/grade 4 OU, anterior chamber depth (ACD) is 3.5 mm OD and 3.6 mm OS, and endothelial cell count is normal OU. Her corneal topography shows:

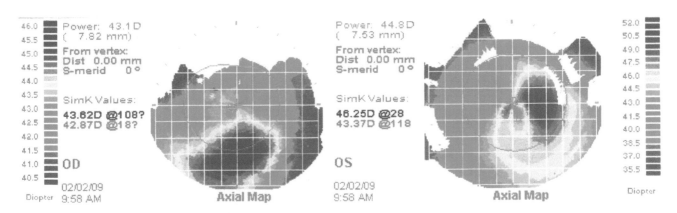

3. How do you interpret the topography maps, and how do the new data affect her surgical options?
4. What are the complications of phakic IOL implantation?

1. Depending on her refractive error, her options include: new glasses with high-index lenses, contact lenses, and refractive surgery. It would be important to know more about her ocular history and exam. Specifically, when did she start wearing glasses, when was her last prescription change, has she tried contact lenses, and if so what type, for how long, and what did she think about them? Does she have any other past ocular history? Has her vision changed recently? How do the glasses interfere with her lifestyle, daily activities, and hobbies? Has she thought about refractive surgery and, if so, what does she hope to accomplish? With regard to the eye exam, what is her current prescription, visual acuity with correction and manifest refraction? Are there any abnormalities on exam?

2. Possible surgical options are laser vision correction, phakic IOL, and RLE. However, the disadvantages of RLE are the loss of accommodation and greater risk of vision-threatening complications due to more invasive surgery. To assist in deciding which option is most appropriate, it is necessary to obtain corneal topography, pachymetry, gonioscopy, ACD, and endothelial cell evaluation.

3. The computerized videokeratoscopy reveals forme fruste keratoconus OD and mild pellucid marginal degeneration OS, and her corneas are thin, so she is not a candidate for laser vision correction. Her surgical options are lens procedures: phakic IOL or RLE. Since she has a stable refraction and excellent vision with glasses at age 38 years old, it is unlikely that her corneas will change significantly. If she desires phakic IOL surgery, a toric design should be considered to correct her astigmatism OS since corneal astigmatic procedures (corneal-relaxing incisions and laser vision correction) should not be performed. However, a small amount of residual ametropia could possibly be corrected with PRK, particularly after corneal collagen cross-linking. Similarly, if she prefers RLE, then toric presbyopia-correcting lenses or toric monofocal IOLs set for monovision should be considered, otherwise she will require glasses for the presbyopia or astigmatism. Multifocal IOLs are usually not a good choice in eyes with this type of abnormal corneal topography because the irregular corneal astigmatism may cause some degree of natural multifocality, increases the unpredictability of IOL calculations, and precludes postoperative keratorefractive surgical enhancement to correct residual ametropia. However, if the irregular astigmatism is mild, is regular/symmetric centrally, the visual acuity is not reduced, and the patient is happy with a multifocal SCL trial, then a presbyopia-correcting IOL can be considered.

4. The main risks are corneal endothelial cell loss, glaucoma, iritis, and cataract. The risk of these complications varies depending on the style of IOL:

   Angle-supported: highest risk of corneal endothelial damage; may also develop glaucoma.

   Iris-supported: highest risk of iris damage, iritis, and IOL dislocation.

   Posterior chamber: highest risk of cataract and angle-closure glaucoma.

   Furthermore, there is a small risk of lens decentration/dislocation, infection, cystoid macular edema, retinal detachment, and disruption of the anterior lens capsule.

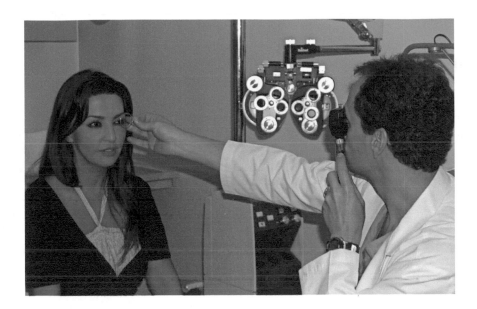

A 34-year-old woman broke her glasses and wants a new prescription. She does not have any old records or glasses to measure.

1.   Describe the technique of streak retinoscopy.

2.   What methods can be used for an irregular cornea?

1. Retinoscopy is a method of objectively measuring the refractive state of an eye. With a phoropter or free lenses, the examiner moves the light streak across the pupil and changes the correcting lenses until the reflex movement is neutralized (pupil appears uniformly illuminated). This occurs at the far point. If the far point is between the examiner and patient (myopic), the reflex moves in the direction opposite to the retinoscope sweep ("against" motion). If the far point is behind the examiner (hyperopia), the reflex has "with" motion. The final refraction is then determined by adjusting for the working distance (add reciprocal of working distance to the final finding).

2. For a scissoring reflex, which occurs in keratoconus, observe the central area of the reflex. If the reflex is poor or irregular, then alternate methods should be used, such as a contact lens overrefraction or stenopeic slit refraction.

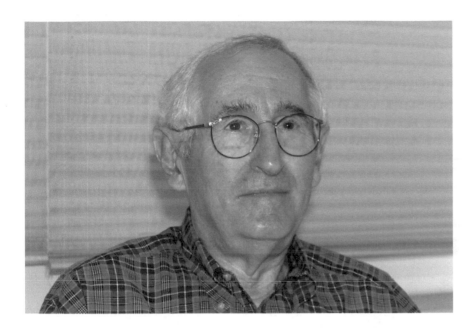

A 73-year-old man reports blurry vision, especially in his right eye. He says he was told he has cataracts but wants a second opinion about surgery. His old glasses are –3.00 +0.75 × 180 OU, and he says he used to have equal vision in both eyes. On exam, you find his manifest refraction is –6.25 +2.00 × 15 OD and –5.00 +1.00 × 180 OS giving BSCVA of 20/70 OD and 20/25 OS. There is a 4+ nuclear sclerotic/2+ posterior subcapsular cataract OD and a 4+ nuclear sclerotic cataract OS. The rest of the eye exam is normal.

1. What additional information would be helpful?
2. How would you advise this patient regarding cataract surgery?

1. More information about the history and symptoms would be helpful: How long has he been having trouble with his vision? How does the reduced vision interfere with his activities (ie, reading, driving, watching TV, computer work, hobbies, glare/halo/starbursts, etc.)? What are his activities/hobbies and how has he used glasses or contact lenses in the past?

    Results of pinhole vision and PAM for OD, and glare test (BAT) for OS would be helpful for determining visual potential OD and visual significance of the cataract OS.

2. This patient has a visually significant cataract OD and possibly one OS, and he also has a large myopic shift with anisometropia. The main issues regarding surgery are the desired refractive outcome and timing of surgery OS.

    Refractive outcome: it is important to inquire about the patient's visual needs and preferred use of glasses for various distances. Since he was a low myope, he may like to read or do close work without glasses and does not mind wearing glasses for driving, so he may prefer a monofocal IOL targeted for reading vision. On the other hand, he may have always found glasses a nuisance and would like to reduce his dependence on them as much as possible, so he may prefer multifocal/EDOF/accommodating IOLs or monovision. Therefore, the various IOL options must be discussed thoroughly.

    Timing of surgery OS: it is also necessary to inform the patient about potential problems with anisometropia/aniseikonia and how this can be addressed with a contact lens if he does not want cataract surgery OS shortly after OD, particularly if he desires full distance correction with cataract surgery OD.

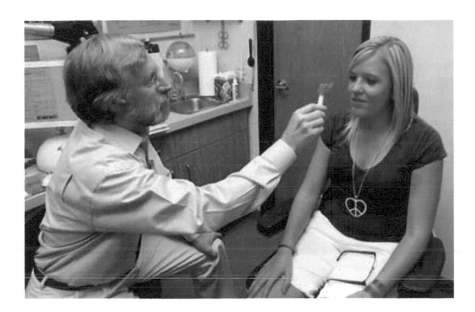

A 23-year-old graduate student complains of headache and eyestrain for the past year. She says her vision has always been fine, but a few years ago she was prescribed a pair of reading glasses. They helped only a little, so she wore them occasionally but lost them after a year. Her past ocular history is otherwise unremarkable.

1. What is the differential diagnosis and how would you determine the diagnosis?

Additional information: she has no past medical history and is not taking any medicines. Her manifest refraction is plano OU, cycloplegic refraction is +0.50 D OU, extraocular motility is full, the eyes are orthophoric at distance and there is a 6 PD exophoria at near, accommodative amplitude is normal.

2. What is the diagnosis?
3. How would you treat this patient?

1. The differential diagnosis includes hyperopia, accommodative insufficiency, and convergence insufficiency. Accommodative insufficiency is associated with systemic processes such as hypothyroidism, anemia, pregnancy, nutritional deficiencies, and chronic illness, so she should be questioned about her past medical history and current medications. The relevant parts of the eye exam to distinguish among the possible etiologies are: manifest and cycloplegic refractions, ocular alignment and motility, near and far points, accommodative and convergence amplitudes. Hyperopia would be revealed by the refractions (other tests would be normal), and convergence insufficiency would be diagnosed by exophoria greater at near than distance.

2. Convergence insufficiency.

3. Orthoptic exercises to improve fusional amplitudes, such as pencil push-ups, may be helpful. Another option is base-out prism glasses to stimulate convergence. Rarely is surgery (medial rectus resection) required.

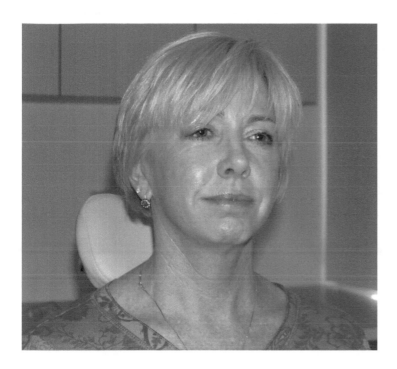

A 51-year-old woman underwent retinal detachment repair with scleral buckle of the right eye 2 weeks ago. Her macula was not affected. She notices that her vision is blurry and she is seeing double. Her uncorrected visual acuity is 20/60 OD and 20/20 OS.

1. What is the most likely cause of her complaints?
2. What single test would help determine the etiology?

Additional information: pinhole improves her vision to 20/20 OD, but does not resolve the diplopia. Her manifest refraction is −2.25 +0.75 × 135 OD and plano OS. She has a right exotropia of 8 PD and hypertropia of 3 PD.

3. How would you manage her?
4. What is the definition of a PD?
5. How are deviations measured with plastic prisms and with glass prisms?
6. How does a minus lens affect the measurement of a tropia?

1. The blurry vision is most likely due to induced myopia (and possible astigmatism) from the scleral buckle, but could be a result of damage from the retinal detachment. The diplopia may also be due to the induced ametropia, but could be caused by strabismus from the scleral buckle.

2. Pinhole vision. If the vision improves, then the blurriness is due to a refractive error. If the diplopia improves, then this is also related to the blurry vision and ametropia. If the diplopia does not improve, then an ocular misalignment is present.

3. She should be given her full glasses prescription with prism correction to alleviate the diplopia. Strabismus surgery or buckle removal could be considered in the future.

4. The displacement (in cm) of a light ray passing through a prism, measured 100 cm (1 m) from the prism.

5. Plastic prisms are held with the back surface parallel to the frontal plane. Glass prisms are held in the Prentice position with the back surface perpendicular to the visual axis. The apex of the prism is pointed in the direction of the eye deviation (ie, base-in for exotropia). Stacking prisms is not additive, but holding prisms in front of each eye is.

6. Minus measures more. Minus lenses make the deviation appear larger; plus lenses decrease the measured deviation. The prismatic effect of glasses on strabismic deviations is calculated as follows: $2.5 \times D = \%$ difference.

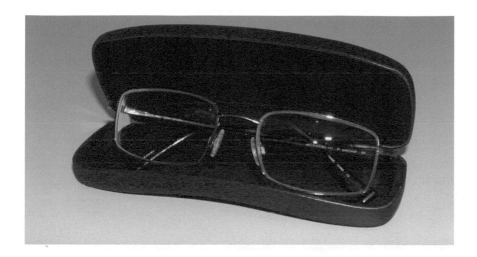

An angry patient walks into your office complaining that the new distance glasses you prescribed are terrible. He has tried them for 2 weeks and cannot get used to them. The glasses make him feel sick. There was only a minor change (0.25 D) in the prescription compared with his old glasses.

1. What do you do?

Additional information: the glasses were made correctly; he says his vision is clear when he looks straight ahead, but everything seems more magnified and his vision is distorted when he looks to the sides; he cannot do anything to make it better. The PD is right, the optical centers are placed correctly, and repeat refraction is the same as the prescription you recently gave him.

2. What else should you check and how?

1. It is important to explain to the patient that there are a number of reasons why he may be having difficulty with the glasses and you will take care of the problem. First, the glasses should be measured with a lensometer to determine whether they were made correctly. If they were, the patient should be questioned about his symptoms: is the vision clear or blurry, is there any distortion, is the difficulty in one eye or both eyes? Can he make it better by adjusting the glasses or moving or turning his eyes or head? Check the ocular alignment of the lenses and repeat the manifest refraction.

2. The base curve of the lenses should be checked with a Geneva lens clock because a change in base curve can cause these symptoms (distortion and the feeling of motion sickness when looking off-center). Increasing the base curve also results in thicker lenses, and more magnification occurs.

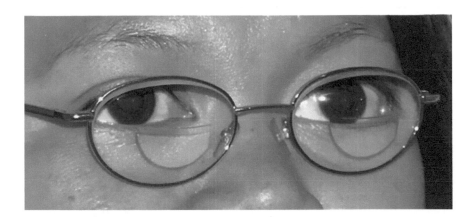

A 16-year-old aphakic girl is interested in wearing contact lenses instead of aphakic glasses. Her manifest refraction is +10.50 +1.00 × 90 OD and +11.25 +0.50 × 90 OS.

1. What are the disadvantages of aphakic spectacles?
2. What would the image magnification be with a contact lens, and with an IOL?
3. What are her contact lens options?
4. Would the power of the contact lenses she requires be stronger or weaker than her glasses prescription? Why?

1. The disadvantages of aphakic glasses are: image magnification of 25%, altered depth perception, pincushion distortion, ring scotoma (prismatic effect at edge of lens causes visual field loss of 20%), and the "jack-in-the-box" phenomenon (peripherally invisible objects suddenly appear when gaze is shifted).

2. There would be 7% image magnification with contact lens and 2.5% with IOL.

3. She could wear soft lenses (spherical OU or possibly a toric lens OD for sharper vision) or RGP lenses OU (which will provide sharper vision by correcting her astigmatism).

4. Because of the difference in vertex distance between glasses and contact lens, the power of the required correcting lens is different. The effectivity of a plus lens increases as it moves further from the eye (greater plus power), whereas the lens effectivity of a minus lens increases as it moves closer to the eye. The more powerful the lens, the more significant is the change in position. As any lens moves closer to the nodal point of the eye, more plus power is required to keep the image focused onto the retina. Therefore, the contact lens this patient needs has more plus power than her glasses lens. The power is determined from:

   1. Focal point of original lens = far point.

   2. Distance of new lens from far point = required focal length of new lens.

   3. Power of new lens = reciprocal of new focal length.

   This can be approximated with the formula: $D2 = D1 + S(D1)2$ (where S = vertex distance in meters).

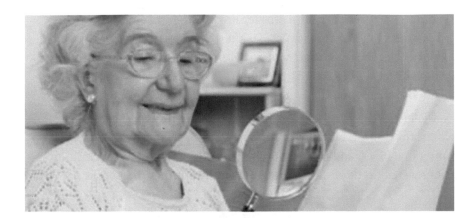

A 76-year-old woman with macular degeneration reports more difficulty with her vision over the past few months. She used to be able to read large print books with bright light but is struggling to do so now, so she wants to get new reading glasses. Her visual acuity is 20/400 OD and 20/80 OS. She denies any change in appearance of the Amsler grid, which she checks several times a week OS. Exam of the maculas shows a disciform scar OD and drusen with RPE atrophy OS.

1. How would you estimate the add power for reading glasses?
2. What type of low-vision aids would be helpful for this patient?

1. Kestenbaum's rule can be used to estimate the strength of the plus lens required to read newspaper print without accommodation. This is useful in patients with low vision. The necessary add power is the reciprocal of the best distance acuity. This patient has no central vision OD and uses her left eye for reading. Therefore, she would need a reading add of +4.00 D (ie, 80/20) for a working distance of 0.25 m (the reciprocal of the add power). This should be checked and refined with trial frames or a phoropter.

2. If the new reading glasses are not sufficient, then other options include spectacle-mounted magnifiers (telescopes for distance or microscopes for near), handheld or stand magnifiers and telescopes, video magnifiers (CCTVs), electronic reading machines, and talking appliances. The patient may benefit from a low-vision consultation to assess her visual needs and try various aids to determine what works best for her.

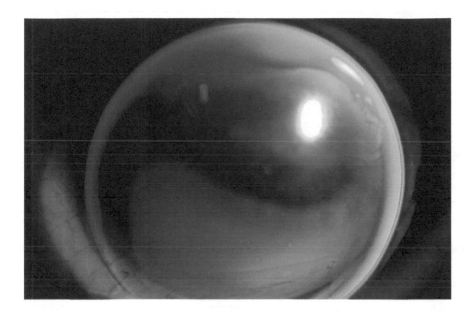

A 53-year-old woman is unhappy with her current contact lenses and wants to be fitted for new lenses.

1. What is the technique for fitting RGP contact lens?
2. What is the technique for fitting SCL?
3. The RGP lens rides high; how can the lens parameters be changed to improve the fit?

1. RGPs are fitted using the "steeper add minus, flatter add plus" (SAM-FAP) rule. The contact lens is fitted steeper than the average corneal keratometry measurement. This forms a plus tear meniscus between the cornea and RGP lens, which alters the required power of the lens. Therefore, it is necessary to subtract power (add minus) at the end of the power calculation. For each diopter the base curve is made steeper than K, subtract 1 D from the final lens power. If the lens is fit flatter than K, then a minus tear meniscus is formed, so it is necessary to add plus power at the end of the calculation. A contact lens overrefraction is performed to determine the necessary power. If a trial lens is not available for overrefraction, then the power calculation is performed as follows:

   - Measure refraction and keratometry.
   - Choose base curve steeper than flat K (usually +0.50 D steeper to form a tear lens; tear lens prevents apical touch).
   - Convert refraction to minus cylinder form and zero vertex distance; disregard the cylinder (minus cylinder is formed by the tears).
   - Power of contact lens is sphere from refraction adjusted for tear lens (subtract +0.50); "SAM-FAP."

   To evaluate the fit, assess the fluorescein pattern, lens movement, and centration.

2. The power of SCL is based on the spherical equivalent manifest refraction corrected for vertex distance. The base curve is based on average keratometry measurements. To evaluate the fit, assess the movement of the lens. Poor movement means the lens is too tight (too steep) and excessive movement indicates that the lens is too flat.

3. The lens is too tight, so to loosen it either increase the radius of curvature or decrease the diameter.

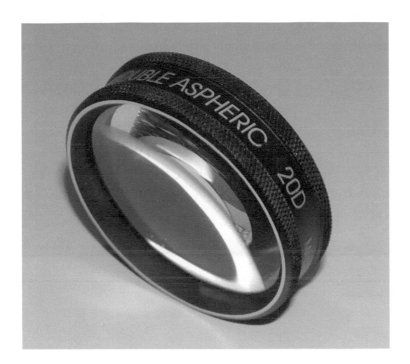

Condensing lenses are used with an indirect ophthalmoscope to examine the retina.

1. What are the advantages of the indirect ophthalmoscope?
2. What are the different types of magnification?
3. What is the retinal magnification with a 20 D lens?

1. Larger field of view and stereopsis compared with the direct ophthalmoscope. Field of view is 25 degrees (versus 7 degrees) and magnification is approximately 2–3× depending on the lens (versus 15×).

2. Transverse, axial, and angular magnification.

    Transverse (linear or lateral): magnification of image size (away from the optical axis). Equal to the ratio of image height to object height ($M_L = I/O$).

    Axial: magnification of depth (along the optical axis). Equal to the square of the transverse magnification ($M_{AX} = M_L^2$).

    Angular: magnification of angle subtended by an image with respect to an object. Used when the object or image size cannot be measured. ($M_A = D/4$, standardized to 25 cm [¼ m], the near point of the average eye.)

3. $M_A = D_{eye}/D_{lens} = 60/20 = 3×$.

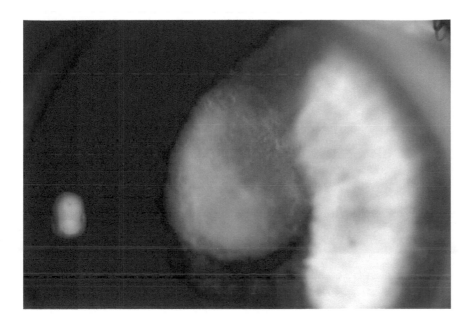

A 34-year-old man with a corneal scar and BSCVA of 20/100 in his right eye wants to know if his vision can be improved.

1. How would you evaluate him?
2. If this patient has better visual potential, what are the surgical options?

1. A number of tests can be performed to determine the visual potential including pinhole acuity, RGP contact lens overrefraction, and PAM test. VER could also be performed.

2. Depending on the location, size, and depth of the scar, the options are PTK, rotational corneal autograft, penetrating keratoplasty, and ALK (superficial [SALK] or deep [DALK]).

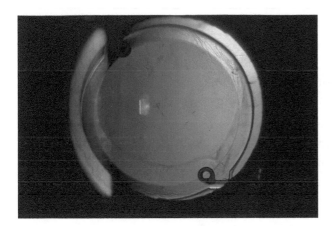

A 68-year-old man sees you for a second opinion. He complains of blurred vision since having cataract surgery 2 months ago. On exam, his uncorrected vision is 20/100 at distance and J1 at near in the operated eye. He is unhappy because he expected good distance vision without glasses and would like to wear glasses to read.

1. What is the problem?

2. What history and findings would be helpful?

3. What are the possible etiologies?

Additional information: old records reveal a history of myopia (−7.50 D), RGP contact lens wear until age 46 when he had LASIK surgery OU. Corneal topography shows:

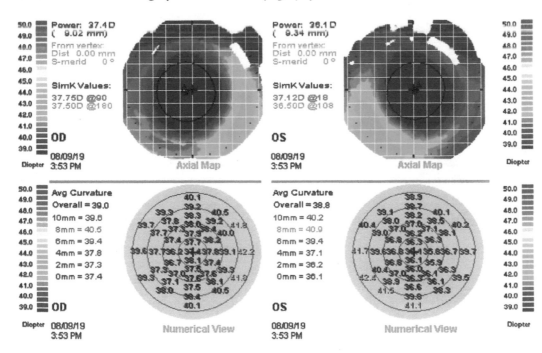

4. What is the most likely cause of his refractive surprise?

5. What are the surgical treatment options?

1. Myopic refractive outcome.

2. The patient should be asked about previous use of glasses/contact lenses, magnitude of prescription, ocular surgery (ie, refractive and retinal procedures) or injuries. Old records are valuable if available. Helpful exam findings include incisions or scarring from previous surgery or trauma, integrity of the capsular bag, IOL position and stability, status of the macula and peripheral retina, and signs of myopic fundus.

3. A refractive surprise after cataract surgery occurs because the IOL is the wrong power or is in the wrong position. Wrong IOL power is due to an error in AL measurement, error in keratometry measurement, use of an incorrect IOL calculation formula, or insertion of the wrong IOL. Wrong IOL position is due to sulcus placement without reducing the IOL power, and anterior displacement of an IOL in the bag from a large capsulorhexis, capsular distension/capsular block syndrome, capsular contraction, or upside-down placement of an angulated IOL.

4. Corneal topography shows a well-centered myopic LASIK ablation with very flat keratometry readings, which is a significant factor in IOL calculation error. There is often a wide range of IOL formula results, which makes choosing the correct IOL power difficult. Intraoperative wavefront aberrometry is helpful in eyes with previous corneal refractive surgery.

5. This patient can be treated with IOL exchange, piggyback IOL, and laser vision correction. For capsular block syndrome, a Nd:YAG laser anterior capsulotomy should be performed to release the trapped fluid and allow the IOL to return to its normal position.

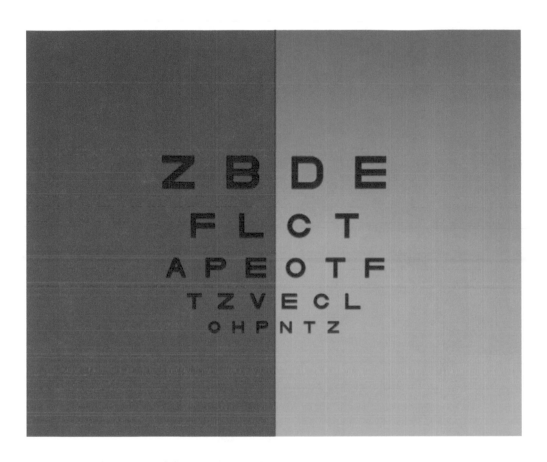

1. What is the name of the test depicted in the photo?

2. How does this test work and how is it performed?

1. The duochrome test.

2. The duochrome test uses the principle of chromatic aberration to monocularly refine the spherical endpoint and check the accuracy and balance of the refraction. Light of shorter wavelengths is refracted more than light of longer wavelengths (green is bent more than red and is therefore focused anterior to red). The green and red filters create a 0.5 D difference. The patient must therefore have 20/30 or better visual acuity in order to distinguish the difference. If the patient sees the letters on the green side of the chart clearer, then the focal point is behind the retina (the eye is overminused) and plus sphere is added to the prescription. If the patient sees the red side clearer, then the focal point is in front of the retina (the eye is overplussed) and minus sphere is added to the prescription. This can be remembered with the mnemonic **RAM-GAP**: Red Add Minus - Green Add Plus. The technique is to start with the red side clearer and add minus sphere in 0.25 D steps until the letters on the red and green sides are of equal clarity (ie, the red and green light are the same distance (0.25 D) behind and in front of the retina, respectively), then the focal point is on the retina and the prescription is balanced. The duochrome test works in colorblind patients because it uses chromatic aberration, not color discrimination.

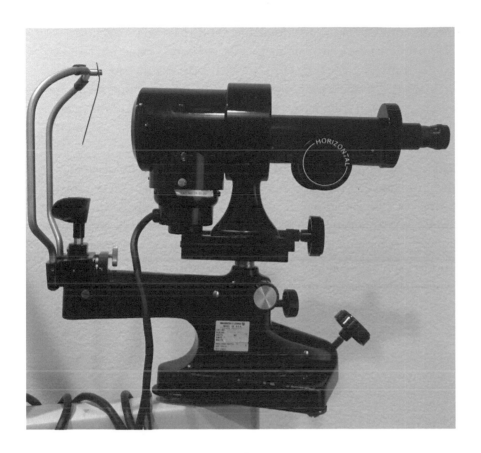

1. What device is shown and how does it work?

2. What are the limitations of this device?

3. What is the astigmatic effect from the posterior corneal surface?

1. A keratometer. This device measures the curvature of the anterior corneal surface based on the power of a reflecting surface. It does this by measuring the size of an image reflected from 2 paracentral points and utilizes doubling prisms to stabilize the image enabling more accurate focusing. The anterior corneal curvature is then calculated using the convex mirror formula, and the corneal power is estimated empirically based on Snell's law of refraction with simplified optics. The keratometer adjusts the index of refraction (1.3375 versus 1.376) to account for the posterior corneal power and also to allow 45 D to equal 7.5 mm radius of curvature (K [diopters] = 337.5/r).

2. Limitations of the keratometer include: it only measures a small region of the cornea (2 points at the 3–4 mm zone), it does not provide information about the cornea central or peripheral to these points, it measures different regions for corneas of different powers, it assumes the cornea is spherocylindrical and symmetric with a major and minor axis separated by 90 degrees, it ignores spherical aberration, it is susceptible to focusing and misalignment errors, and it cannot accurately measure irregular corneas.

3. The posterior corneal surface contributes approximately 0.4 D of against-the-rule astigmatism to the total corneal power. This is important when determining the amount of corneal astigmatic correction during cataract surgery and RLE.

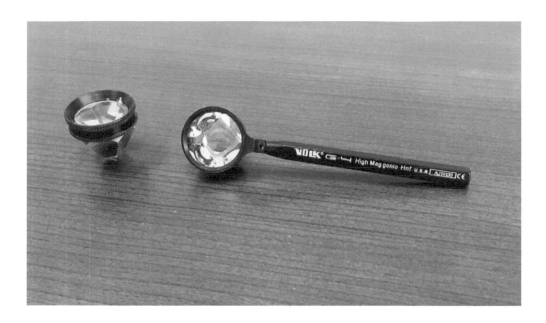

1. Name the various types of gonioscopy lenses and explain how they differ.

2. Define the critical angle.

3. What is total internal reflection and how is this relevant to the eye exam?

1. There are a variety of gonioscopy lenses: Koeppe-style lenses (ie, Koeppe, Barkan, Wurst, Swan-Jacob, and Richardson) for direct gonioscopy (direct and upright view of the iridocorneal angle structures with a binocular microscope, light source, and supine patient, usually in the operating room), and the Goldmann-style lenses and the 4- or 6-mirror lenses (ie, Zeiss, Posner, Sussman) for indirect gonioscopy (indirect and inverted view of the opposite angle with the slit lamp biomicroscope and patient sitting upright).

   The Goldmann lenses typically contain three mirrors, but there are lenses with only one mirror. The lens rests on the sclera, vaults over the cornea and therefore requires a viscous coupling solution (ie, Goniosol), and cannot be used for indentation gonioscopy. In the three-mirrors lenses, each mirror has a different angulation to view different parts of the eye: the angle (~60 degrees), peripheral retina (~65 degrees), and mid-peripheral retina (~75 degrees). The center of the lens can be used to visualize the posterior pole. Because only one of the mirrors can be used for angle viewing, the lens must be rotated 360 degrees to examine the entire angle.

   The 4- and 6-mirror lenses are composed of symmetric mirrors with the same angulation (~60–63 degrees) so that the angle structures can be viewed with minimal or no rotation of the lens. These lenses rest on the cornea without the need for a coupling solution. This enables the examiner to perform indentation gonioscopy to differentiate between appositional and synechial angle closure. Appositional angle closure opens with indentation of the central cornea, which pushes aqueous peripherally, and synechial angle closure does not open with indentation.

2. The critical angle is the angle at which incident light is bent 90 degrees away from the normal (when going from a medium of higher to lower index of refraction, n) and after which all light is reflected. The critical angle differs for different interfaces and depends upon the indices of refraction of the material on either side of the interface. The critical angle of the cornea (air/cornea interface) is 46.5 degrees.

3. Total internal reflection is an optical phenomenon that occurs when the angle of incidence exceeds the critical angle. This causes light to be reflected back into the material with higher index of refraction. Angle structures cannot be directly visualized owing to total internal reflection at the air/cornea interface. Therefore, a gonioscopy lens is required to view the angle structures.

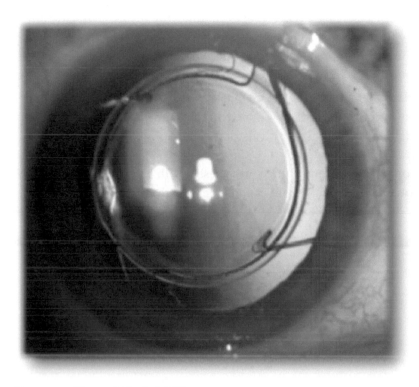

(Courtesy of Samuel Masket, MD)

A 72-year-old woman has a +2.00 D refractive surprise after cataract surgery and desires a piggyback IOL procedure.

1. How is the correct piggyback IOL power calculated, and what power does this patient require for emmetropia?
2. What are the necessary considerations when planning to perform a piggyback IOL procedure?

1. As a general guideline, to correct myopia the necessary IOL power is 1.2 times the myopic refractive error, and to correct hyperopia the necessary IOL power is 1.5 times the hyperopic refractive error. The Holladay R formula can also be used to calculate the appropriate power for a piggyback IOL. In this case, a +3.00 D IOL should be used to achieve emmetropia.

2. The relevant considerations for piggyback IOL procedures are the IOL power, material, edge design, and position. IOLs with low negative or low positive dioptric power are required. The material should be different from that of the existing IOL in the eye (ie, acrylic versus silicone) to minimize the risk of an intralenticular membrane formation. The piggyback lens is placed in the ciliary sulcus and should have a rounded (not square) edge, a posterior angulation, and a three-piece design with sufficient overall length in order to prevent pigment dispersion and iris damage from chafing the posterior iris surface.

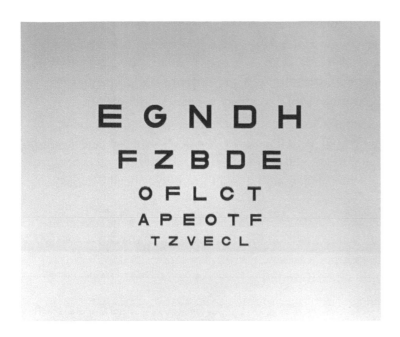

1. What is Snellen acuity, and what does Snellen notation mean?
2. What are the characteristics of the ETDRS chart?

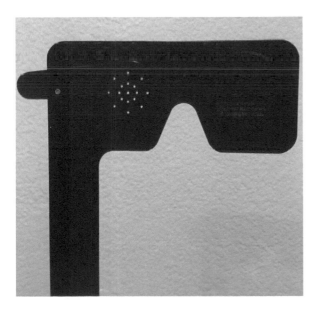

3. What is the principle of a pinhole?
4. What is the optimal size of a pinhole and why?

1. Snellen acuity refers to the standard 20/20 notation of measuring visual acuity and is based on the angle that the smallest letter subtends on the retina. The numerator refers to the testing distance (ie, 20 feet or 6 meters); the denominator represents the distance at which a letter subtends 5 minutes of arc (ie, 20/40 letter subtends 5 minutes at 40 feet, 20/20 letter subtends 5 minutes at 20 feet), or the distance at which a person with normal vision can see the letters. Each stroke width and space subtends 1 minute of arc.

2. The ETDRS visual acuity measurement was designed to eliminate the inaccuracies of other tests and is considered the gold standard for population studies and clinical research. The ETDRS chart is characterized by a proportional layout and geometric progression of letter sizes. The chart consists of five letters per line, the space between letters is equal to the size of the letters on that line, and the optotype height changes in 0.1 log unit increments.

3. A pinhole allows only the undeviated paraxial light rays to focus on the retina. It reduces refractive error and improves vision by increasing depth of focus, but it is limited by diffraction. A pinhole can correct for up to 3 D of refractive error and can also improve vision in eyes with corneal or lenticular irregularities. However, a pinhole can reduce vision in eyes with retinal disorders.

4. The optimal size of a pinhole is 1.2 mm. A smaller hole limits visual acuity because of increased diffraction and reduced amount of light entering the eye.

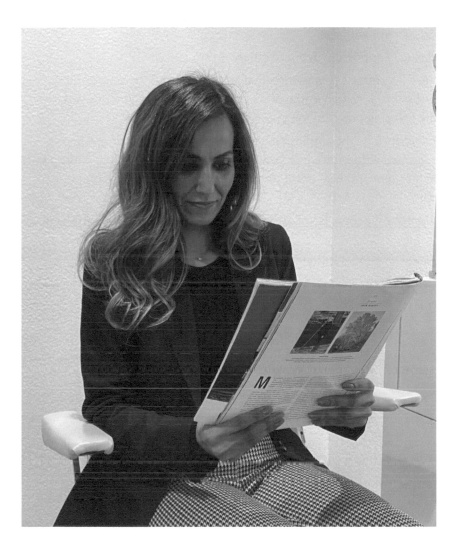

A 47-year-old woman with low myopia complains of trouble reading the newspaper. She wears contact lenses less frequently and has to take off her glasses to read.

1. What is the problem?
2. What is the pathogenesis?
3. Explain the Helmholtz theory of accommodation.
4. How is accommodation measured?
5. What is the differential diagnosis of premature presbyopia (subnormal accommodation)?
6. Explain Donder's table.

1. Presbyopia, the natural loss of accommodation with age.

2. Presbyopia is caused by loss of lens elasticity or possibly reduced ciliary muscle effectivity.

3. During accommodation, the ciliary muscle contracts (parasympathetic innervation) decreasing zonular tension on the capsule allowing the crystalline lens to become more convex (mainly the anterior surface) and move forward, which increases the focusing power of the eye.

4. The accommodative response can be described by the amplitude of accommodation (total dioptric amount the eye can accommodate; measured with Prince rule [see Case 3] or method of spheres) or range of accommodation (distance between far point and near point of the eye; measured with tape measure or accommodative rule).

5. Debilitating illness, head injury, CN3 palsy, Adie tonic pupil, drugs (tranquilizers), diphtheria, botulism, mercury toxicity.

6. Donder's table shows the average accommodative amplitudes for different ages.

   Up to age 40: accommodation decreases by 1 D every 4 years (starting at 14 D at age 8).

   At age 40: accommodation is 6 D (±2 D).

   Between age 40 to 48: accommodation decreases by 1.5 D every 4 years.

   After age 48: accommodation decreases by 0.5 D every 4 years.

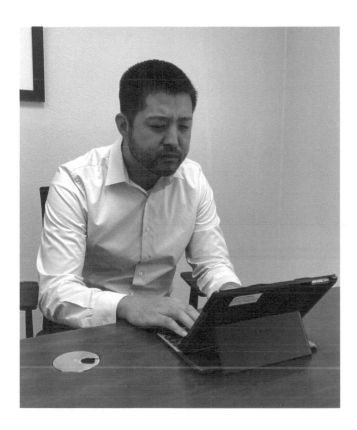

A 34-year-old man reports blurry vision and headaches when working on the computer for more than 20 minutes. He had a prescription for reading glasses in graduate school but never used them. On exam, his uncorrected vision is 20/20 in each eye at distance and J2 at near. Manifest refraction is plano OD and −0.25 sphere OS. His near vision improves to J1+ with +1.25 sphere OU. The rest of the examination is normal.

1. What is the patient's problem?
2. What is asthenopia, and what conditions are associated with it?
3. What test would be most helpful?
4. How would you treat the refractive error?
5. What are the surgical methods for correcting hyperopia?
6. What is the prevalence and natural history of this condition?
7. What is the differential diagnosis of acquired hyperopia?

1. Hyperopia with asthenopia. As the patient ages, he is no longer able to accommodate to fully compensate for all of his hyperopia, and therefore he is experiencing asthenopia.

2. Asthenopia refers to the symptoms of eye strain (ocular pain, fatigue, headache, blurry vision, light sensitivity) with sustained near effort (from ciliary muscle contraction during accommodation). Most commonly, this is caused by uncorrected presbyopia, pre-presbyopic hyperopia, and overminused myopia. Other etiologies include extraocular muscle imbalance, improper lighting, hypothyroidism, anemia, pregnancy, nutritional deficiencies, and chronic illness.

3. Refraction. A cycloplegic refraction to reveal the total amount of hyperopia, and later, a careful postcycloplegic refraction pushing plus in a trial frame (to allow the patient to adapt) to determine the prescription that the patient will accept.

4. In general, hyperopes should be prescribed their full hyperopic correction to provide clear distance and near vision, rather than give only reading glasses, which treats the symptom not the underlying condition. However, older hyperopes who have compensated by accommodating, do not wear glasses, and are nearing presbyopic age may prefer not to wear distance glasses and just wear reading glasses. However, with increasing presbyopia, they will eventually require distance glasses (when they can no longer compensate with accommodation).

5. LTK, CK, excimer laser (PRK, LASIK), RLE, and phakic IOL (outside United States).

6. At birth, babies have approximately +3.0 D of hyperopia, which decreases to approximately +1.0 D by the age of 2 years. In children, the prevalence of hyperopia ($\geq$ +2.0 D) is inversely associated with age, declining from almost 8.5% at the age of 6 years to approximately 1% at 15 years. The frequency is higher in Caucasians and those living in rural areas. Hyperopia ($\geq$ +0.50 D) prevalence is ~30% in adults and is associated with increasing age (approximately 20% in the 5th decade of life and 60% after the 8th decade of life).

7. *Decreased effective AL*: retrobulbar tumor, choroidal tumor, central serous chorioretinopathy, posterior scleritis, serous retinal detachment.

   Decreased refractive power: lens change (posterior lens dislocation, aphakia, diabetes), drugs (chloroquine, phenothiazines, antihistamines, benzodiazepines), poor accommodation (tonic pupil, drugs, trauma), corneal flattening (contact lens, RK surgery), intraocular silicone oil.

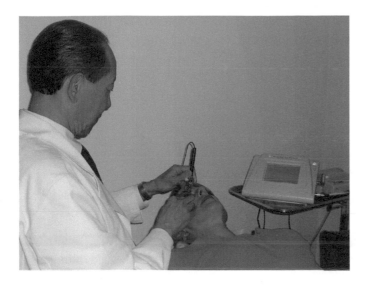

1. What type of device is depicted, and what does it measure? What alternative method can be used?

2. What measurements are necessary for calculating IOL power?

3. How are IOL formulas classified, and what are the advantages of the newer ones?

4. Why are IOL calculations challenging after keratorefractive surgery?

1. A-scan ultrasound to measure AL prior to cataract surgery. Partial coherence interferometry (ie, IOLMaster, Lenstar) measures AL and also provides other ocular dimensions and IOL calculations.

2. Corneal curvature and AL.

3. *First generation*: ACD is constant.

   Second generation: ACD based on AL.

   Third generation: (Holladay 1, Hoffer Q, SRK/T) ACD based on AL and K.

   Fourth generation: (Holladay 2) variables include AL, K, corneal diameter, ACD, lens thickness, refraction, and patient age; (Haigis) ELP derived from a function instead of a single number.

   Fifth generation: (Olsen, Barrett Universal II) used in IOLMaster and Lenstar devices; (Hoffer H-5) based on Holladay 2 and racial variations.

   Other: (Hill-RBF) pattern recognition algorithm; (Ladas super formula) amalgam of existing formulas.

   The newer formulas are more accurate. Most accurate third and fourth generation formulas according to AL:

   - Short eyes (<22.0 mm): Hoffer Q and Holladay II
   - Medium eyes (22.0–24.5 mm): Hoffer Q, Holladay I or 2, SRK/T, Haigis
   - Medium-long eyes (24.5–26.5 mm): Holladay 1 or 2
   - Long eyes (>26.5 mm): SRK/T, Holladay 2, Haigis

   The Wang-Koch adjustment formulas improve the accuracy in eyes with AL ≥ 25.2 mm.

4. Corneal refractive surgery changes the anterior corneal curvature in a nonuniform way. This causes less accurate measurements with traditional methods of keratometry, which results in less predictable IOL calculations and refractive outcomes. Correction formulas and intraoperative wavefront aberrometry are helpful for achieving better results.

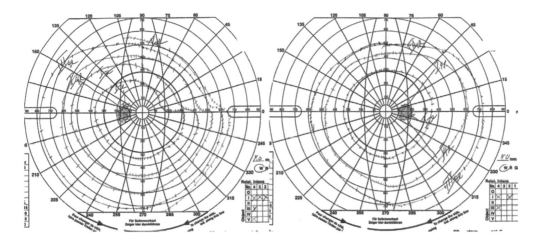

A 60-year-old woman says she needs a pressure check. She has been treated for glaucoma for 3 years with a prostaglandin analog in both eyes. Her vision is 20/25 OU, IOP is 14 mmHg OU, and she has a stable superior arcuate VF defect in the left eye. Her right ON head appears normal and her left ON head is depicted below:

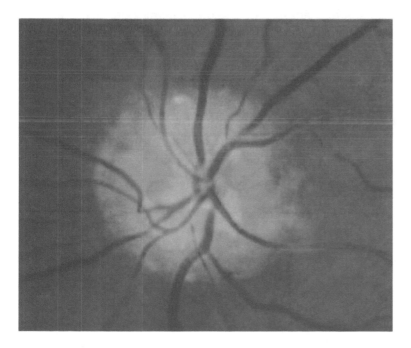

1. What does her ON photo show?

2. What is the pathophysiology?

3. What tests can be used to confirm the diagnosis?

4. What is pseudopapilledema, and what is the differential diagnosis?

5. How would you manage this patient?

6. What are the potential complications of ON drusen?

1. ON head drusen (pseudopapilledema).

2. Superficial or buried hyaline bodies in the prelaminar optic nerve that have become calcified.

3. B-scan ultrasound, CT scan, or autofluorescence.

4. Optic disc elevation without edema. Optic disc drusen (most common), congenital anomalies (hypoplastic optic disc, tilted optic disc, glial tissue, myelinated nerve fibers), small/crowded disc (usually associated with hyperopia), vitreopapillary traction, optic nerve mass or infiltration (neoplastic or inflammatory), peripapillary mass (ie, astrocytic hamartoma), Leber hereditary optic neuropathy, Alagille syndrome.

5. It is important to determine whether this patient's VF defect is due to glaucoma or the ON head drusen. Therefore, it would be helpful to obtain her old records to know what old field tests showed, what her maximum eye pressure was, and whether her ON appearance has changed. If she never had elevated IOP or progression of the scotoma or optic cupping, then the glaucoma diagnosis may be suspect and it is reasonable to stop the glaucoma drop and follow her IOP. A diurnal curve may also be useful for determining her maximum IOP. If previous records are unavailable, then new baselines should be established with visual fields, gonioscopy, corneal pachymetry, and optic nerve head images.

6. Optic nerve drusen can cause VF defects (typically enlarged blind spot, arcuate scotoma, or sectoral scotoma that is stable/nonprogressive). Rare complications include anterior ischemic optic neuropathy, choroidal neovascularization, subretinal or vitreous hemorrhage, and vascular occlusion.

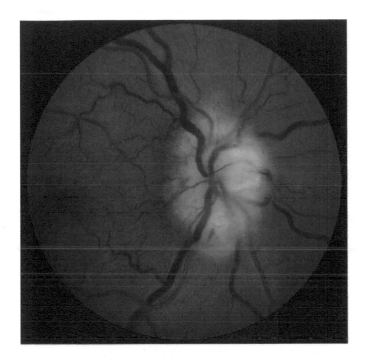

A 70-year-old man reports intermittent double vision for the past week and is panicked because of blurry vision in the right eye for 2 days. He says his vision has been excellent since his cataract surgery several years earlier. He takes medication for hypertension and high cholesterol. Ocular exam shows visual acuity of 20/200 OD and 20/25 OS. There is a positive RAPD in the right eye, extraocular motility is full, and anterior segment exam reveals well positioned posterior chamber intraocular lenses. The retina is within normal limits and the right ON is pictured above.

1. What are you concerned about and what further history would you obtain?
2. How would you work up this patient?
3. What treatment would you prescribe if this patient has GCA, and what is the prognosis?
4. What is Foster–Kennedy syndrome and pseudo-Foster–Kennedy syndrome?

1. The history and findings are suggestive of AION. It is important to distinguish between the arteritic (GCA, 5%) and non-arteritic (NAION, 95%) forms because the arteritic form must be treated to prevent visual loss in the fellow eye. NAION has an unknown etiology but is associated with hypertension, diabetes, ischemic heart disease, hypercholesterolemia, and smoking. This patient has increased blood pressure and cholesterol, but it cannot be assumed that his optic neuropathy is nonarteritic. The patient must be asked about the characteristic symptoms of GCA: headache, scalp tenderness, jaw claudication (pain with chewing), weight loss, fever, and anorexia, as well as neck pain, eye pain, diplopia, joint pain (symptoms of polymyalgia rheumatica), and history of anemia.

2. A stat ESR, sed rate is required to rule out arteritic AION. An elevated ESR is considered to be > (age/2) for males and > ([age + 10]/2) for females. Other labs that should be ordered are (elevated CRP [>2.45 mg/dL]) and CBC (low hematocrit, high platelets). Fluorescein angiography shows choroidal nonperfusion in the arteritic form. Some physicians routinely obtain a temporal artery biopsy (sometimes bilateral) on all patients, which should be performed within 2 weeks of initiating steroid treatment. Because of skip lesions, the biopsy specimen should be at least 3 cm in length.

3. Emergent treatment with high-dose steroids (prednisone 60–120 mg orally; consider IV initially [1 g qd for 3 days]), which should not be delayed while waiting for the temporal artery biopsy. Unfortunately, treatment does not improve the outcome in the affected eye but is necessary to prevent visual loss in the fellow eye (65% risk of involvement without treatment; however, some patients lose vision despite treatment). Patients should be followed by an internist and/or rheumatologist to monitor the response to therapy and to slowly taper the steroids. GCA is also associated with other ocular and systemic complications: retinal artery occlusion, ophthalmic artery occlusion, anterior segment ischemia, cranial nerve palsy (especially CN 6), and stroke.

4. Foster–Kennedy syndrome is a frontal lobe mass (usually meningioma) that causes anosmia, ipsilateral optic atrophy from tumor compression, and contralateral optic nerve edema from elevated intracranial pressure. The same optic nerve findings (disc edema in one eye and disc pallor in the other eye) can occur in bilateral AION, which is called pseudo-Foster–Kennedy syndrome.

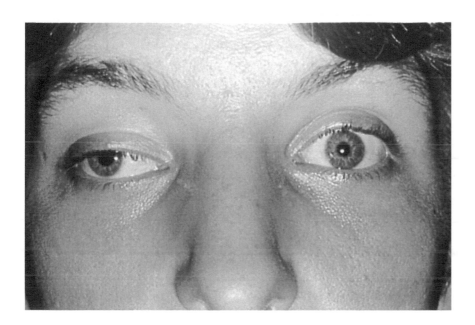

A 45-year-old woman reports double vision that started this morning after breakfast. She also notices that her eyelid seems droopy. She has mild hypertension and says her blood pressure has been stable for years on medication.

1. What findings are seen in the photo?
2. What other history would you ask the patient?

Additional information: the patient says that she has a headache but she often gets headaches, although this seems worse and has not improved significantly with ibuprofen. She denies any trauma. On exam, her vision is 20/20 OU, there is a right upper eyelid ptosis, and the right eye is turned down and out. The right pupil is large and poorly reactive to light. Other cranial nerves are intact. Intraocular pressure is 18 mmHg, and the rest of the anterior and posterior segment exams are normal.

3. What are the diagnosis and possible etiologies?
4. What would your next step be?
5. How would your treatment differ if this patient were older than 50 years of age with an isolated pupil-sparing third nerve palsy?

1. This patient has a right upper eyelid ptosis, ocular misalignment, and anisocoria with a larger right pupil.

2. The patient should be asked about headache and a history of trauma or cancer.

3. This patient has a pupil-involving CN 3 palsy OD. Despite a history of hypertension, she is young and has pupil involvement, and pain. It is therefore most important to rule out a posterior communicating artery aneurysm, which is a neurosurgical emergency. It is unlikely to be due to other etiologies such as microvascular (diabetes, hypertension), trauma (no history of this), tumor, or infection.

4. Urgent neuroimaging with MRI, MRA/CTA, or both.

5. Older patients with isolated pupil-sparing third nerve palsies should be observed carefully for pupil involvement during the first week, but generally such cases are due to microvascular disease (80% are pupil sparing) and resolve spontaneously in 3 months. Workup is performed if the pupil becomes involved, there is a history of cancer, there are other neurologic abnormalities, signs of aberrant regeneration are present, or the palsy does not resolve after 3 months. The diplopia can be treated by occluding the paretic eye.

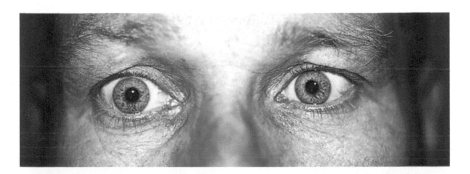

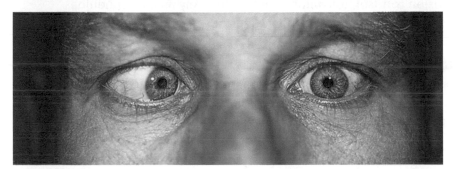

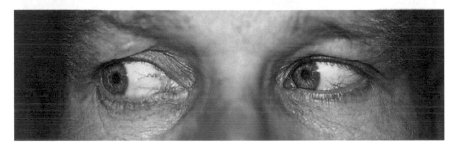

A 55-year-old man reports double vision for a week. He wears bifocals and has had no other change in vision. Exam shows 20/30 vision, normal pupillary responses, mild cataracts, and normal posterior segments in both eyes. Results of ocular motility testing are depicted in the photo.

1. What abnormality does this patient have?
2. What are the possible etiologies?
3. What additional history is pertinent?

Additional information: this is the first time he has had double vision. His past ocular history is negative. He does have diabetes, which is controlled with oral medication.

4. What workup and treatment are required?

1. The patient has an esotropia in primary gaze and deficiency of abduction OS. This is consistent with a lateral rectus (CN 6) palsy.

2. Most commonly it is vasculopathic in adults, but other etiologies include trauma, temporal arteritis, infection, multiple sclerosis, cerebrovascular accidents, increased intracranial pressure, and, rarely, tumors. Other conditions in the differential diagnosis of CN 6 palsy are thyroid eye disease, orbital pseudotumor (idiopathic orbital inflammatory disease), myasthenia gravis, convergence spasm, strabismus, medial orbital wall fracture, and orbital myositis.

3. Has he ever had previous episodes of diplopia or neurologic symptoms? Any previous eye problems, surgery, or trauma? Is the double vision constant, intermittent, or variable? Any medical conditions, specifically hypertension, diabetes, cancer? Any weakness, fatigue, difficulty breathing/swallowing, hoarseness?

4. Treatment of CN 6 palsy depends on the underlying etiology. This is presumably an ischemic isolated mononeuropathy due to diabetes, which is self-limited and should resolve within 3 months, so a workup is not necessary. The patient should be reassured and told that he can temporarily cover his left glasses lens or patch the left eye to prevent diplopia or use prism glasses. He should be monitored for other neurologic symptoms. If any develop or his condition does not resolve in 3 months, then neuroimaging is indicated. Additional workup to consider is checking BP, lab tests (CBC, ESR, VDRL or RPR, FTA-ABS or MHA-TP ANA), lumbar puncture, and Tensilon test.

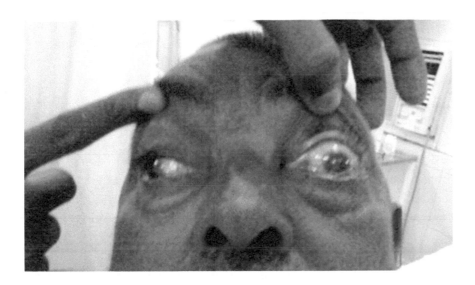

A 64-year-old man presents to the ER with left-sided facial pain, swollen eyelid, and double vision. He is a low myope with no significant past ocular history. His visual acuity is 20/40 OD and 20/60 OS without correction and extraocular motility in the left eye is restricted in all positions of gaze.

1. What is the differential diagnosis?
2. What other exam findings might be present?
3. How would you work up this patient?

Additional information: the patient's visual acuity with correction is 20/20 OU, there is no RAPD or efferent defect, but he does have anisocoria with a miotic left pupil. He also has a left ptosis, ocular motility is limited in all positions of gaze, and there is decreased facial sensation of the left forehead and cheek.

4. What nerves are involved and where is the pathology?

1. This patient appears to have multiple CN palsies. These can be caused by tumor, infection, inflammation, meningitis, and vascular lesions in the brain stem, subarachnoid space, cavernous sinus, or orbital apex. Other disorders that mimic multiple CN palsies include CPEO, myasthenia gravis, multiple sclerosis, Guillain–Barré syndrome, and progressive supranuclear palsy.

2. Depending on the location of the pathology, other cranial nerves and sympathetic nerves may be affected, so a CN exam must be performed with particular attention to BCVA, anisocoria, pupillary response, extraocular motility, lid position, facial sensation, and facial muscle strength. Possible findings include decreased visual acuity and color vision (orbital apex syndrome), ptosis, strabismus, negative forced ductions, decreased facial sensation in CN V_1–V_2 distribution, relative afferent pupillary defect, miosis (Horner syndrome), and trigeminal (facial) pain. There may also be proptosis, conjunctival injection, chemosis, increased intraocular pressure, bruit, and retinopathy in cases of high-flow arteriovenous fistulas. Fever, lid edema, and signs of facial infection occur in cases of cavernous sinus thrombosis.

3. Head, orbital, and sinus imaging (CT/MRI–MRA) is required to localize the pathology and direct treatment. Lab tests to order include fasting blood glucose, CBC with differential, ESR, VDRL or RPR, FTA-ABS or MHA-TP, ANA, and blood cultures if infection is suspected. Other possible tests include lumbar puncture and Tensilon test.

4. The history and findings reveal involvement of CN 3, 4, V_1, V_2, 6, and sympathetics (Horner syndrome), which indicate a cavernous sinus lesion. In contrast, orbital apex syndrome involves CN 2 and does not involve V_2 or the sympathetics (ie, CN 2, 3, 4, V_1, and 6).

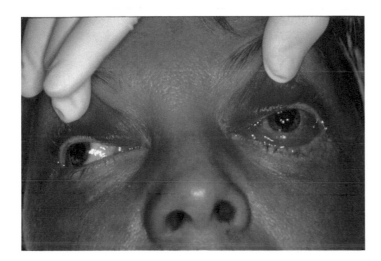

You are called to see a 52-year-old woman in the ER with a 1-week history of progressive periorbital pain, headache, redness, and swelling.

1. What would you ask this patient?
2. What is the differential diagnosis?
3. What would you look for on exam to determine the correct diagnosis?

Additional information: the patient is diabetic and was admitted to the ER with a blood glucose level of 625 mg/dL. She has decreased acuity, proptosis, and limited extraocular motility.

4. What organisms cause this infection, and what are you most concerned about?

Additional information: a biopsy shows:

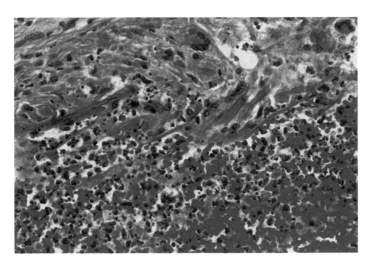

5. What is the appropriate treatment?
6. What are the possible complications?

1. Is there any history of trauma, surgery, bites/scratches, infection (sinus, dental, systemic), diabetes? Any fever? Does she notice a change in vision or diplopia? Does she have pain with eye movement?

2. Preseptal or orbital cellulitis, idiopathic orbital inflammation, thyroid eye disease, subperiosteal abscess, orbital neoplasm (eg, rhabdomyosarcoma, lymphoproliferative disease, ruptured dermoid cyst), orbital vasculitis, trauma, carotid-cavernous fistula, cavernous sinus thrombosis.

3. Preseptal cellulitis is an infection anterior to the orbital septum and does not affect the globe, whereas orbital cellulitis is an infection extending posterior to the septum and involves the globe (therefore has eye findings, specifically decreased vision, positive RAPD, restricted ocular motility, proptosis, pain on eye movement, periorbital swelling, chemosis, and optic disc swelling).

4. Orbital cellulitis is most commonly due to Gram-positive bacteria (*Streptococcus* and *Staphylococcus* species) but can also be caused by fungi (Phycomycetes). Mucormycosis, an aggressive infection by *Mucor* fungi that causes necrosis, vascular thrombosis, and orbital invasion, must be suspected in this case of an immunocompromised patient.

5. This is *Mucor* infection (the histology shows broad nonseptate fungal hyphae and angiothrombosis), a life-threatening condition requiring emergent IV antifungals and surgical debridement. A CT scan should be obtained to evaluate the extent of involvement. The diabetes must be treated and controlled.

6. *Mucor* can cause retinal vascular occlusions and orbital apex syndrome. It may extend intracranially to cause cavernous sinus thrombosis, meningitis, brain abscess, and death.

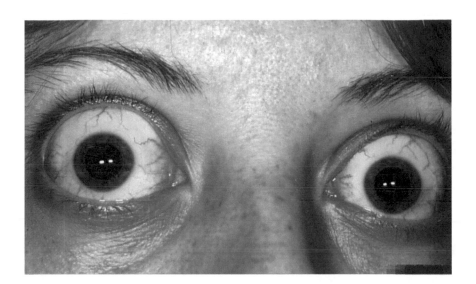

A 28-year-old woman reports that her eyes have been red for the past year and seem bigger.

1. What is the most likely diagnosis?

2. What other ocular findings are associated with this condition?

3. What is the treatment?

4. What are other causes of proptosis in an adult?

5. What tests are helpful in determining the correct diagnosis?

1. TED, usually from Graves' disease, is the most common cause of unilateral or bilateral proptosis.

2. In addition to proptosis, other findings include lid signs (lid retraction, lid lag on downgaze, lagophthalmos), restricted extraocular motility (strabismus), exposure (conjunctival hyperemia, keratopathy), and optic nerve compression (optic neuropathy). The Werner classification of eye findings in Graves' disease can be remembered with the mnemonic **NO SPECS**: **N**o signs or symptoms, **O**nly signs, **S**oft tissue involvement, **P**roptosis, **E**xtraocular muscle involvement, **C**orneal involvement, **S**ight loss (optic nerve compression).

3. TED can be treated with Tepezza. Dry eye is treated with lubrication, patching/taping/goggles at bedtime, punctal occlusion, and sometimes with tarsorrhaphy. Extreme proptosis causing severe keratopathy or optic nerve compression is treated with orbital decompression. Diplopia can be treated with prism glasses and eventually surgery (rectus recessions when the strabismus is stable for at least 6 months). Steroids and sometimes radiation are used to reduce muscle enlargement. Surgery is performed in a stepwise fashion with orbital decompression first, then strabismus surgery, and finally lid surgery (eyelid recession). The underlying thyroid disease must also be treated.

4. The differential diagnosis of proptosis in an adult includes orbital pseudotumor (idiopathic orbital inflammatory disease), orbital and lacrimal gland tumors, orbital vasculitis, trauma, cellulitis, arteriovenous fistula, and cavernous sinus thrombosis.

5. A complete eye exam must be performed with attention to visual acuity, color vision, pupils, motility, forced ductions, eyelid position and movement, exophthalmometry, cornea, tonometry (increased IOP in upgaze), and ophthalmoscopy. Check visual fields as a baseline study in early cases and to rule out optic neuropathy in advanced cases. Thyroid function tests (TSH, thyroxine [total and free T_4], and triiodothyronine [T_3]) and TSI should be ordered. Orbital CT scan may show extraocular muscle enlargement with sparing of the tendons (the inferior rectus is most commonly involved, followed by medial, superior, lateral, and oblique [mnemonic **IMSLO**]), in contrast to IOI, in which the tendons are also enlarged.

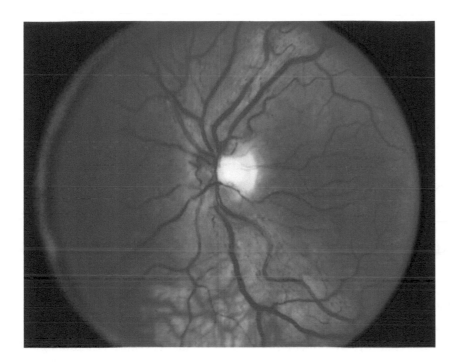

A 24-year-old man reports blurry vision in the right eye and then the left eye gradually for several weeks. He is hyperopic with no past ocular or medical history. His BCVA is 20/400 OD and 20/200 OS; pupillary response, extraocular motility, and intraocular pressure are normal. Anterior and posterior segment exams are essentially normal. The optic nerve appearance is shown in the figure.

1. What other history would be useful?

Additional information: the patient's grandfather has macular degeneration, both grandparents have cataracts, and an uncle had poor vision for most of his life. He takes vitamins but no medications. He is a social drinker and occasionally smokes a cigar. He has no known toxic exposures, and his past medical history is negative.

2. What is the differential diagnosis?
3. What additional tests would you perform?

Additional information: retinal exam is normal, he has centrocecal scotomas, and significant color vision impairment in both eyes.

4. What is the most likely diagnosis?
5. What are the characteristic findings of this disease?
6. What do you tell him about the disease?

1. Is there any family history of eye problems or visual loss (particularly at a young age)? Any medications, alcohol or tobacco use, toxic exposures, or nutritional deficiencies? Does he have a history of infectious diseases or cancer? Any significant radiation exposure?

2. Hereditary or acquired optic neuropathies (compressive, toxic, nutritional, infectious, traumatic, infiltrative, ischemic).

3. Visual fields and color vision testing. Genetic testing for mutations in the respiratory chain complex I genes, MT-ND1, MT-ND4, MT-ND4L, or MT-ND6. MRI to rule out demyelinating disease and compressive lesions. OCT may show peripapillary NFL swelling in acute cases, and diffuse thinning in chronic cases.

4. The most likely diagnosis is LHON.

5. The typical appearance is disc hyperemia, peripapillary telangiectatic vessels, tortuous vessels, peripapillary nerve fiber layer edema, and eventually optic disc pallor. Additional findings include movement disorders, dystonia, tremors, cardiac conduction defects, Leigh syndrome, and MS-like symptoms can be seen in a condition called LHON plus.

6. LHON is a hereditary optic neuropathy that is a mitochondrial disease with maternal inheritance, so it is transmitted to all sons (only 50% are affected; in females 15% are affected). Visual loss occurs in the 2nd to 3rd decade of life with bilateral sequential loss of vision to worse than 20/200. Unfortunately there is no cure. A clinical trial (RHODOS - Rescue of Hereditary Optic Disease Outpatient Study) of 300 mg Idebenone tid, a synthetic form of coenzyme Q10, has shown to be effective in approximately half of cases, but the primary endpoint was not met. The G11778A mutation is most common and associated with most severe disease. The T14484C mutation has the best prognosis with visual recovery seen in some cases. The G3460A mutation has the worst prognosis.

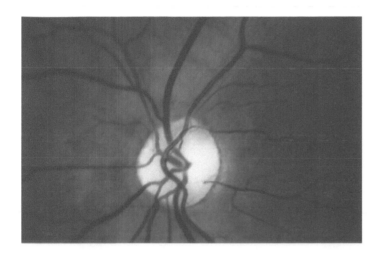

A 56-year-old woman reports progressive decreased vision in her left eye for the past 3 months. Her past ocular history is negative. On exam, her visual acuity is 20/20 OD and 20/100 OS. Extraocular motility is intact, confrontation VF appear full, and there is a positive RAPD in the left eye.

1. What do you notice about the optic nerve?
2. What additional testing would you perform in the office?

Additional information: color vision is normal OD and reduced OS. Her VF shows:

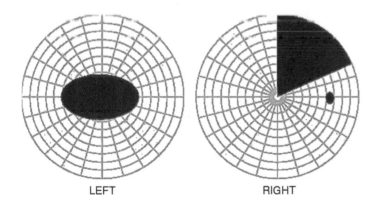

LEFT   RIGHT

3. Does the VF test localize the pathology and, if so, where is the lesion?
4. What is the differential diagnosis?
5. What additional workup is necessary?

1. Optic disc pallor horizontally.

2. VF (tangent screen, Humphrey, or Goldmann) and color vision testing.

3. The VF defect is a junctional scotoma due to a lesion of the optic nerve near the chiasm, which involves the knee of von Willebrand (inferonasal retinal fibers that cross in the chiasm and then travel anteriorly approximately 4 mm into the opposite [contralateral] optic nerve before running posteriorly to the brain) causing central visual loss in the ipsilateral eye and a superotemporal field defect in the contralateral eye.

4. Chiasmal syndrome, which is most commonly a mass lesion but possibly due to hemorrhage. The differential diagnosis includes tumors, pituitary apoplexy, aneurysm, trauma, sarcoidosis, and chiasmal neuritis.

5. Neuroimaging; also consider endocrine evaluation (check hormone levels).

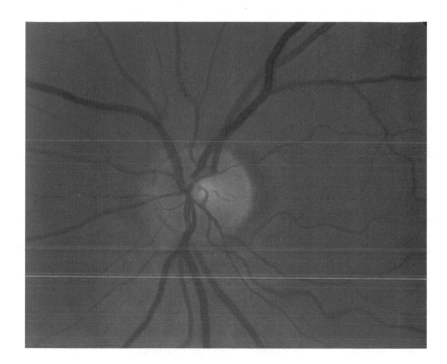

A 33-year-old woman reports decreased vision and eye pain in the left eye that started 2 days ago and has gotten worse. She says everything looks blurry and appears dimmer with that eye.

1. What would you ask this patient?
2. What would you specifically look for on exam?
3. What is the differential diagnosis?

Additional information: she denies any trauma or previous episodes. Her past medical history is negative and she takes only birth control pills. The eye hurts especially when she looks to the right and left. There is no redness, photophobia, or diplopia. She has no other associated symptoms. Her exam is normal, except for 20/200 vision and a positive RAPD OS.

4. What is the diagnosis?
5. What other unusual findings are associated with this disease?
6. What additional testing would you perform and why?
7. What are the recommendations for treatment?
8. What is the prognosis?

1. What type of eye pain (foreign body sensation, sharp, dull, ache, tender to touch, pain with eye movement, headache, periorbital pain)? Any double vision? Any trauma? Any previous episodes? Has the eye been red? Any sensitivity to light? Any other neurologic symptoms? Does she have any medical conditions? Is she taking any medication?

2. On exam, it is important to check the visual acuity, pupillary response with attention to the presence of a RAPD, extraocular motility, cornea, anterior chamber reaction, vitreous, retina, and ON.

3. Corneal lesion (foreign body, abrasion, erosion, ulcer), uveitis, optic neuritis.

4. Retrobulbar optic neuritis.

5. Pulfrich phenomenon (motion of pendulum appears elliptical because of altered depth perception from delayed conduction in the demyelinated nerve), Uhthoff phenomenon (worsening of symptoms with heat or exercise; present in 50% after recovery), and phosphenes (flashes of light induced by eye movements or sound).

6. Check color vision, VF, serum aquaporin-4 autoantibodies (AQP4-IgG; to rule out neuromyelitis optica [Devic disease; optic neuritis (usually bilateral) and transverse myelitis]), and neuroimaging (MRI to look for periventricular white matter demyelinating lesions or plaques (the best predictor of future development of multiple sclerosis) and to look for spinal cord and brainstem lesions of neuromyelitis optica). A neurologic exam should also be performed. In patients with atypical findings (ie, older age, no pain, acute severe or persistent (>1 month) visual loss, bilateral involvement, papillitis with peripapillary hemorrhages, exudates, intraocular inflammation, other cranial nerve involvement) also perform RPR and FTA-ABS (for syphilis); ESR and ANA (for SLE); C-ANCA (for granulomatosis with polyangiitis); Lyme and *Bartonella* titers; ACE, CXR or CT, gallium or PET scan (for sarcoidosis); and consider genetic testing (for LHON).

7. According to the ONTT, if the MRI is positive, then consider systemic steroids (methylprednisolone 250 mg IV q6h for 3 days, followed by prednisone 1 mg/kg/day for 11 days and rapid taper 20 mg/day on day 12 and 10 mg/day on days 13–15). Visual recovery occurred 2 weeks faster with this regimen than with other treatments; however, there was no difference in the final visual acuity. Furthermore, there was a decreased incidence of MS over the next 2 years, but there was no difference after 3 years. Oral steroids should not be used alone owing to an increased risk of recurrent optic neuritis.

8. Most patients recover vision over the following months, but the final acuity depends upon the severity of the visual loss. The majority of patients recover 20/20 vision; however, permanent subtle color vision and contrast sensitivity deficits are common. Uhthoff symptoms (blurred vision with increased body temperature or exercise) may occur. Approximately 30% of patients with isolated optic neuritis will experience another attack in either eye, and up to 50% of patients will develop MS over 5–10 years. Risk of MS is 72% in 15 years if patient has one or more lesions on MRI.

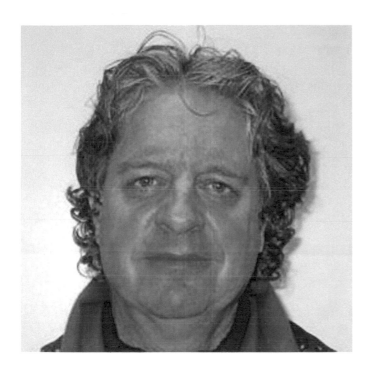

A 57-year-old man complains of recent loss of vision. He is a poor historian and tends to ramble. His vague and inconsistent story makes it difficult to elicit an accurate account of his symptoms, but it appears that the decreased vision was sudden and painless. His eye exam is normal, except for visual acuity of 20/400 OU.

1. What do you suspect may be the problem and what other questions might be helpful?
2. What tests could you perform to confirm your suspicion?

Additional information: you determine that this patient has hysteria.

3. What strategies can you use to help him "recover" his vision?

1. This case is suspicious for functional visual loss (ie, malingering, hysteria). Malingering is the fabrication of a disorder for secondary gain (usually financial), whereas hysteria is a subconscious expression of symptoms. In order to distinguish between them and rule out any organic disease, it would be helpful to ask about any injuries, medical problems, medications, and social history with particular attention to employment status, stresses, and alcohol/drug use.

2. Carefully performing a variety of vision tests to trick the patient can usually uncover functional visual loss because of inconsistent results. These include distance and near, monocular and binocular, varying the test distance, fogging, red–green glasses with duochrome test or Worth four dot test, prism dissociation, stereopsis, startle reflex, proprioception, name signing, mirror tracking, and optokinetic nystagmus response. Visual fields may show unusual patterns such as tunnel vision, spiraling fields, and crossing isopters. Finally, in difficult cases electrophysiologic testing, OCT, fluorescein angiography, or neuroimaging may be necessary.

3. It is helpful to acknowledge the decreased vision and then offer reassurance and a potential way out such as administering a topical medication in the office and then retesting, or having the patient return in several weeks for a repeat examination. Psychiatry consultation is usually not required.

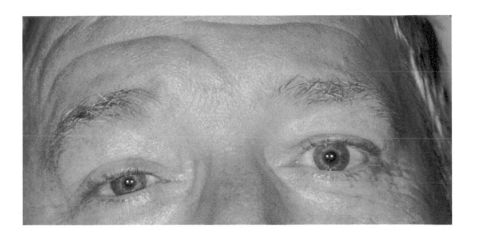

A 58-year-old man presents with a droopy eyelid. He denies any change in vision.

1. What do you notice in the picture?
2. What is the most likely diagnosis?
3. What are the etiologies?
4. What additional history and findings would be helpful?

Additional information: the patient denies any trauma and has no other symptoms. He does not have blurry vision or diplopia. On exam, his vision is 20/20 in both eyes, there is a right upper eyelid ptosis. The eyes are aligned and ocular motility is full. The right pupil is smaller than the left, and there is no relative afferent or efferent pupillary defect. CNs are intact. The rest of the anterior and posterior segment exams are normal.

5. What is the differential diagnosis of anisocoria?
6. What type of pupil testing would you perform?

1. The patient has a right upper eyelid ptosis and anisocoria with a smaller right pupil.

2. Horner syndrome.

3. The etiology depends upon which neuron is affected: central causes include cerebrovascular accident, neck trauma, tumor, cervical disc disease, and demyelinating disease. These rarely result in an isolated Horner syndrome. Preganglionic causes include tumors (mediastinal, apical, thyroid), trauma, pneumothorax, cervical infections, brachial plexus syndromes, carotid artery dissection, aneurysm, trauma. Postganglionic causes include neck lesion, head trauma, migraine, cavernous sinus lesion, vascular lesions (carotid dissection, carotid-cavernous fistula, internal carotid artery aneurysm), and infections. The most common etiologies are idiopathic, internal carotid artery dissection, stroke, surgical, and tumor.

4. How long has he noticed the ptosis? Does it vary? Has he noticed the difference in pupil size? Any change in vision or double vision? Has he had any head or eye trauma? Any pain, headache, or other neurologic symptoms? On exam, what are his visual acuity, pupillary response, and extraocular motility? What does the CN exam show?

5. This depends on whether the abnormal pupil is smaller (ie, greater anisocoria in a dim/dark room) or larger (ie, greater anisocoria in bright light/well-lit room). For a miotic pupil, the differential diagnosis includes Horner syndrome, Argyll Robertson pupil, iritis, and pharmacologic (pilocarpine, brimonidine, narcotics, insecticides). For a mydriatic pupil, the differential diagnosis includes Adie tonic pupil, CN 3 palsy, Hutchinson pupil, pharmacologic (mydriatic, cycloplegic, cocaine, hallucinogen), iris damage (trauma, ischemia, or surgery [Urrets-Zavalia syndrome]). If the anisocoria is equal in light and dark, then the diagnosis is physiologic anisocoria (difference in pupil size ≤ 1 mm).

6. Pharmacologic testing for Horner syndrome consists of two steps:

   1. Topical cocaine 4%–10% to determine the presence of Horner syndrome: if there is increased anisocoria (after 40 minutes), then Horner syndrome exists (if the pupillary dilation is equal, then the diagnosis is simple anisocoria).

   2. Topical hydroxyamphetamine 1% (Paredrine) to distinguish between preganglionic and postganglionic lesions: if the dilation is equal, then Horner syndrome is central or preganglionic; if the dilation is asymmetric then Horner syndrome is postganglionic.

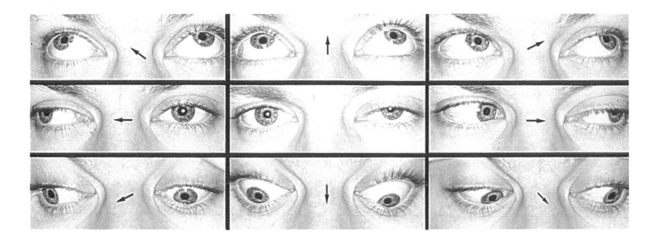

A 49-year-old woman reports droopy eyelids for the past 6 months and is interested in surgery. She says sometimes she has to raise her lids to keep her eyes open. Her vision seems to be unchanged, but occasionally when driving she notices that the line on the road is double, especially when she looks to her right. She wears bifocal glasses and has no other past ocular history.

1. What is the differential diagnosis of transient diplopia?

2. What additional history would be helpful?

Additional information: the patient is suspected of having MG.

3. What are the characteristic eye findings of this disease and what tests would be useful for confirming the diagnosis?

4. What other workup and treatment are necessary for this disease?

1. The most common causes of transient diplopia are decompensated phoria, convergence or divergence insufficiency, MG, and spasm of accommodation. Other etiologies include GCA (EOM ischemia), vertibrobasilar insufficiency, superior oblique myokymia, cyclic esotropia, and skew deviation.

2. Is the ptosis worse on one side, does it vary (ie, throughout the day, from day to day, when she is tired)? Has she ever had diplopia before? Does it happen with other activities such as reading, watching TV, etc.? Is it associated with a headache or other neurologic symptoms? Has she had any eye or head trauma? Any other medical problems, specifically autoimmune disorders? Any weakness, difficulty in breathing or swallowing, hoarseness?

3. The characteristic ocular findings of MG are asymmetric ptosis and variable strabismus. Gaze-evoked nystagmus also occurs. There is no pupil or ciliary muscle involvement. The hallmark of the disease is variability and fatigability, so there is worsening of the ptosis with extended upgaze and improvement with rest or cold. This can be evaluated with the rest test (improvement in ptosis after closing the eyes for 30 minutes) or ice test (improvement in ptosis after application of an ice pack for 2 minutes). Forced ductions are negative. A Tensilon test can be administered to observe for improvement in ocular signs; however, a negative test does not rule out MG. The diagnostic lab test is ACh receptor antibodies. If these tests are negative, then definitive diagnosis is by single fiber EMG of peripheral or orbicularis muscles.

4. It is important to rule out thyroid disease, thymoma, and other autoimmune disorders, so lab tests (thyroid function tests, ANA, and RF) and a chest CT or MRI scan should be obtained. The patient should be referred to a neurologist or internist for systemic treatment. Strabismus can be managed with prism spectacles and potentially surgery when stable for at least 6 months.

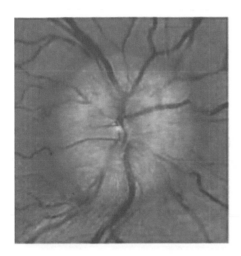 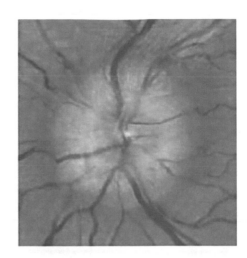

A 32-year-old woman complains of diplopia for several weeks. She has also had headaches for months. On exam you find an obese, slightly anxious woman with vision of 20/25 in both eyes, normal pupillary response, and esotropia in primary gaze. The optic nerve appearance is shown.

1. What is the abnormality?
2. What is the differential diagnosis?
3. What other tests would you perform in the office?
4. What is the workup for papilledema, and how do you determine whether she has IIH?

Additional information: the patient has IIH.

5. What are the associations?
6. What is the treatment?
7. What is the most likely cause of her diplopia?

1. Bilateral optic disc swelling.

2. Papilledema (intracranial mass, infection, infiltration, hemorrhage, or IIH [pseudotumor cerebri]), malignant hypertension, diabetic papillitis, or compressive optic neuropathy (TED, IOI), pseudopapilledema.

3. Check the pupils for RAPD, color vision, visual fields, extraocular motility (consider forced ductions), lid position and presence of proptosis, and resistance of the globes to retropulsion. The patient's blood pressure must be checked to rule out hypertension. She should also have a serum blood glucose level.

4. Neuroimaging and LP. IIH is a diagnosis of exclusion that is determined by four criteria:

    1. Signs and symptoms of increased intracranial pressure (ie, headache, vomiting, papilledema).

    2. High cerebrospinal fluid pressure (>250 mmH$_2$O) with normal composition.

    3. Normal neuroimaging studies.

    4. Normal neurologic examination except for possible CN 6 palsies.

5. IIH is associated with medications (steroids [use or withdrawal], oral contraceptive pills [due to hypercoagulability and dural sinus thrombosis], vitamin A, tetracycline, nalidixic acid, lithium, and isotretinoin), chronic obstructive lung disease, dural sinus thrombosis, radical neck surgery, recent weight gain, and pregnancy.

6. Any medication associated with IIH should be discontinued, and a weight loss regimen should be instituted for obesity. Patients with vision loss, VF defects, or intractable headaches are treated with systemic medications (acetazolamide [Diamox] or furosemide [Lasix]). Patients with progressive visual loss may require surgery (ON sheath fenestration, lumbar-peritoneal shunt).

7. CN 6 palsy.

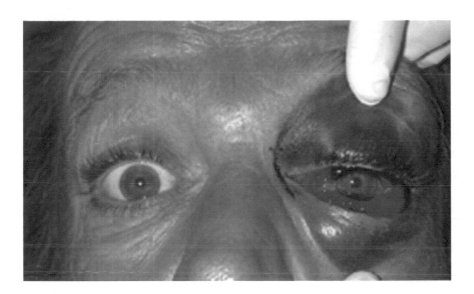

A 48-year-old man reports being hit by an elbow in his left eye while playing basketball last night. He complains of pain, swelling, and sensitivity to light. Exam of the left eye reveals a visual acuity of 20/40, limited supraduction, and an external exam as noted in the photo. There is subconjunctival hemorrhage and anterior chamber cells and flare. The posterior segment is normal.

1.　What would you expect to see on orbital CT scan?
2.　What other signs may be present?
3.　What bones comprise the orbit?
4.　What are the most common sites of fracture?
5.　How would you treat this patient?
6.　What are the indications for surgery?
7.　If this patient were a child, how would the management differ?

1. The presentation is consistent with an orbital floor fracture with entrapment, which should be evident on orbital CT scan. This is the most common type of orbital fracture, and usually involves the maxillary bone and the posterior medial floor, the weakest point of the orbit.

2. Other signs of a blowout fracture are globe ptosis, infraorbital nerve hyperesthesia, and lid emphysema.

3. *Roof*: frontal, sphenoid (lesser wing)

    Lateral wall: zygomatic, sphenoid (greater wing)

    Floor: maxillary, palatine, zygomatic

    Medial wall: ethmoid, lacrimal, sphenoid (body of), maxillary

4. Orbital wall fractures occur in isolation or with displaced or nondisplaced orbital rim fractures. The floor is most common (usually posterior maxillary bone) and then the medial wall (usually lacrimal and ethmoid bones).

5. Initially, the patient should be treated with ice compresses, nasal decongestants, and avoid blowing his nose. Consideration should be given to prescribing oral antibiotics and steroids for 10 days. He also has a traumatic iritis, which should be treated with a topical steroid and cycloplegic. He should be reevaluated for surgery in 7–10 days to allow for reduction of swelling.

6. The indications for repair are diplopia, muscle entrapment, enophthalmos, and facial asymmetry.

7. Pediatric floor fractures are different from those in adults because the bones are pliable and a trapdoor situation may occur, in which the inferior rectus or surrounding tissue can become entrapped. Nausea and bradycardia occur owing to the oculocardiac reflex. This is commonly referred to as a "white-eyed blowout fracture" because the eye is usually quiet; however, it requires emergent surgery to prevent permanent damage to the entrapped tissue.

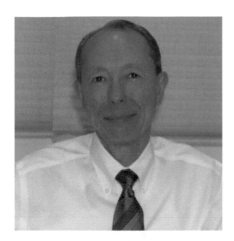

A 63-year-old man reports difficulty in reading. He says that the words are clear, but he has trouble following the lines of text and loses his place. He denies any change in vision, headaches, or other neurologic symptoms. Exam shows visual acuity of 20/20 in both eyes at distance and near, normal pupillary response without a RAPD, early cataracts, and normal fundus exam.

1. What other tests would you perform?

Additional information: extraocular motility is full and the eyes are orthophoric. Amsler grid reveals a blurry area inferotemporal to fixation in the right eye. Humphrey VF testing shows:

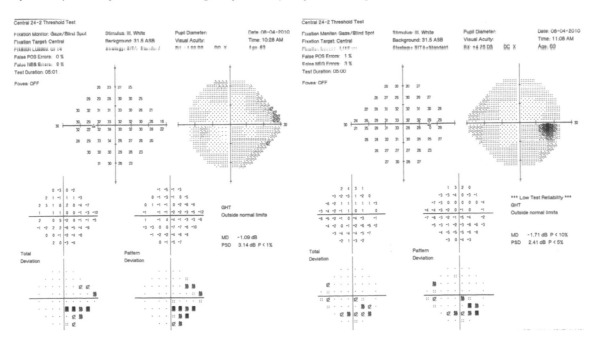

2. What does the VF test show?
3. Where is the pathology?
4. What would you do next?

1. Extraocular motility including alternate cover testing, Amsler grid, and VF.

2. The VF reveals right homonymous inferior quadrantic scotomas.

3. This indicates a lesion involving the left parietal lobe.

4. Obtain neuroimaging, which should be coordinated with the patient's internist.

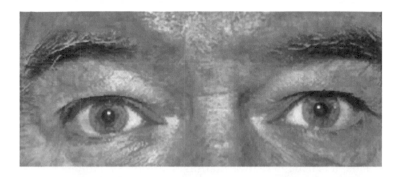

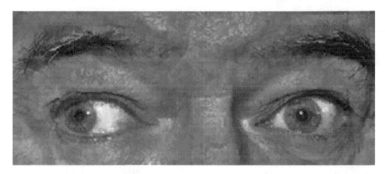

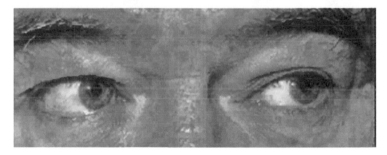

A 50-year-old man complains of double vision beginning 2 days ago.

1. What do the photos demonstrate?
2. What is the differential diagnosis?
3. What exam findings would be helpful to determine the diagnosis?

Additional information: the patient does have contralateral abducting nystagmus, but no ptosis or other motility limitations.

4. What is the diagnosis?
5. Where is the lesion?
6. What are the etiologies?
7. What are the signs of bilateral involvement?
8. How does this differ from one-and-a-half syndrome?

1. Horizontal gaze palsy with an inability to adduct the left eye.

2. Internuclear ophthalmoplegia, medial rectus palsy, myasthenia gravis.

3. The presence of other neurologic signs, contralateral abducting nystagmus (INO), absence of convergence (anterior INO), absent doll's head maneuvers and caloric stimulation (INO), ptosis (MG), other extraocular motility limitations (MG), variability/fatigability (MG).

4. INO.

5. MLF.

6. The etiology depends on age. In patients <50 years, it is usually demyelination or tumor. In patients >50 years, it is usually vascular. Other causes are trauma, infection, and compression.

7. Inability to adduct either eye, impaired convergence, appearance of exotropia in primary gaze.

8. One-and-a-half syndrome is due to a lesion of the PPRF or CN 6 nucleus, and the ipsilateral MLF. This causes ipsilateral gaze palsy and INO, so the only eye movement present is abduction of the contralateral eye with nystagmus. Etiologies include stroke, MS, basilar artery occlusion, and pontine tumors.

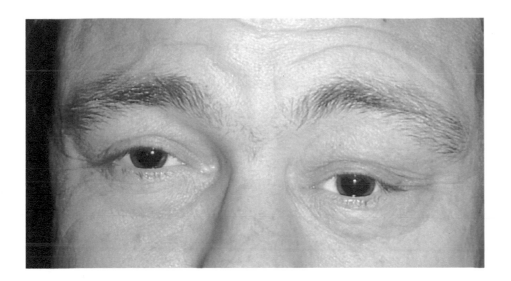

A 61-year-old man complains of double vision for the past month.

1. What abnormality is present in the photo?
2. What are the differential diagnosis and most likely diagnosis?

1. Globe dystopia with the left globe displaced inferiorly.

2. Globe dystopia is caused by a mass lesion. The differential diagnosis of adult orbital tumors is large, but the most common tumors are cavernous hemangioma, meningioma, neurilemmoma, fibrous histiocytoma, lymphoid lesion, lacrimal gland and sinus tumors, and metastases. Patient age, direction of globe displacement, and presence or absence of pain help to narrow the diagnosis. Most lesions are intraconal masses that cause proptosis. Lacrimal and sinus tumors typically cause the globe to be displaced inferiorly. In this case, the patient's left eye is being pushed down and out, which is probably due to a sinus mucocele, most commonly from the frontoethmoid sinus.

Additional information: a CT scan is obtained to confirm the diagnosis.

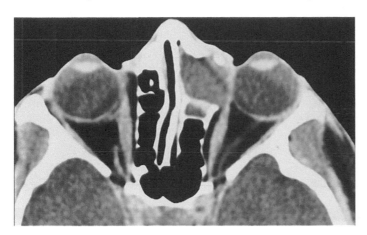

3. Describe the findings. What is the diagnosis?

4. What is the treatment?

5. If instead the CT scan showed a well-circumscribed fusiform tumor, and the histopathology appeared as in the figure below, what would be the diagnosis?

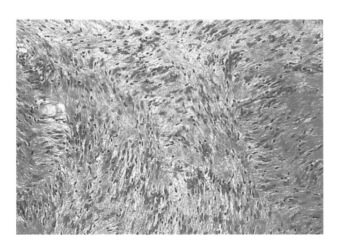

3. The CT scan shows opacification of the left anterior ethmoid sinus with erosion into the orbit. This represents a sinus mucocele.

4. Surgical excision and IV antibiotics.

5. The figure demonstrates the typical arrangement of spindle cells in an Antoni A-pattern neurilemmoma.

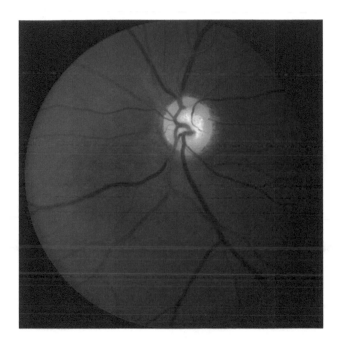

A 46-year-old man complains of poor vision for years. On exam, his BSCVA is 20/200 OU, color vision and contrast sensitivity are decreased, the cup-to-disc ratio is normal and there is optic disc pallor OU.

1. What other history would you like to know?

Additional information: the patient reports a gradual deterioration of his vision over the last 6 years but cannot be more specific. Although he suffered several sports-related concussions in college, he denies any ocular trauma or eye disease and is unaware of any family history of eye problems except for cataracts. His only medication is a statin for high cholesterol, although he does have a history of taking multiple antibiotics after a positive PPD skin test. He works as a bartender and admits to recreational drug use and struggling with alcohol abuse in the past.

2. What is the differential diagnosis?
3. What testing would you perform?

Additional information: VF testing shows bilateral central scotomas; MRI of the head and orbits is normal.

4. What diagnosis do you suspect?
5. What are the causes of toxic optic neuropathy?
6. What are the causes of nutritional optic neuropathy?
7. How would you manage a patient who is taking ethambutol?

1. It is important to obtain a complete past medical and ocular history, medication history, family history, and social history, with specific attention to any factors that can contribute to optic nerve damage. Specifically, does the patient have a history of any eye disorders, trauma, surgery, systemic disease with ocular manifestations, malignancy or infectious disease, major blood loss, radiation treatment, or using medications with ocular toxicity? Is there any hereditary eye disease in the family? What are his alcohol, drug, tobacco and nutrition habits? It would also be helpful to know about the timing and progression of the visual loss and how it affected each eye.

2. Optic neuropathy: hereditary, compressive, infiltrative, infectious, toxic, nutritional, traumatic, or retrobulbar.

3. VF exam and CT or MRI scan to rule out compressive or infiltrative etiology.

4. Toxic or possibly nutritional optic neuropathy.

5. Ethambutol is the most common; others include isoniazid, rifampin, chloramphenicol, streptomycin, sulfonamides, methanol, ethylene glycol, arsenic, lead, digitalis, chloroquine, quinine, linezolid, imipramine, cisplatin, busulfan, vincristine, disulfuram, cyclosporine, methotrexate, lead, mercury, thallium, carbon monoxide, and tobacco-related or alcohol-related amblyopia. Ischemic-like optic neuropathy can occur with phosphodiesterase 5 inhibitors (sildenafil, vardenafil, tadalafil) and amiodorone.

6. Vitamin deficiencies: B1 (thiamine), B2 (riboflavin), B6 (pyridoxine), B12 (cobalamin), and folic acid.

7. Ethambutol toxicity depends on dose and duration (after 2 months of use the incidence is 1% for 15 mg/kg/day, 6% for 25 mg/kg/day, 18% for > 35 mg/kg/day); other risk factors are age > 65 years old and hypertension. For high risk patients (taking > 15 mg/kg/day, long duration, vitamin deficiency, renal failure) monitor central vision monthly with visual acuity, color vision, visual field, Amsler grid, and consider contrast sensitivity and OCT (RNFL) testing. A complete eye exam is indicated for any visual changes. There are no guidelines for patients on lower doses, but a reasonable follow up interval is 3 months. With early detection of ethambutol optic neuropathy (visual changes without optic atrophy), 30%-64% of patients regain vision (~2 Snellen lines) after stopping the medication.

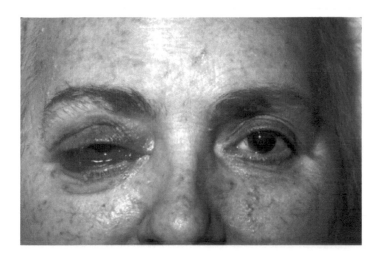

A 58-year-old woman complains of pain and swelling of her right eye for the past month, with increasing redness over the last week.

1. What is the differential diagnosis?
2. What other history would be helpful?

Additional information: she has double vision but denies any fever, nausea, vomiting, or recent trauma or infection. She has hypertension, which is well controlled with an oral medication. She is otherwise healthy and has not had similar symptoms in the past.

3. How would you work up this patient?

Additional information: exam shows restricted extraocular motility with positive forced ductions OD. Palpation of the lids and globes demonstrates fullness of the right upper eyelid laterally and resistance to retropulsion. Proptosis is present by Hertel exophthalmometry. Anterior and posterior segment exams are normal except for conjunctival injection and chemosis. The IOP is normal. Thyroid function tests are normal. CT scan shows an enlarged lacrimal gland and extraocular muscle enlargement with involvement of the tendons.

4. What is the most likely diagnosis?
5. What is the treatment?
6. What is Tolosa–Hunt syndrome?

1. The differential diagnosis for ocular pain, eyelid edema and erythema, and conjunctival injection and chemosis includes trauma, orbital cellulitis, vasculitis, tumor, arteriovenous fistula, cavernous sinus thrombosis, and thyroid eye disease.

2. Has she noticed a change in vision or double vision? Has she had any ocular trauma or surgery? Any recent infection? Does she have any systemic diseases, particularly autoimmune disorders or cancer? Has she had any previous episodes?

3. Complete eye exam with attention to visual acuity, pupillary response, extraocular motility, proptosis, lid/adnexal masses, cornea (sensation, exposure), intraocular pressure, anterior chamber reaction, and optic nerve appearance (disc edema). Consider thyroid function tests. Orbital CT or MRI scan to rule out mass, abscess, and evaluate muscles/tendons.

4. Idiopathic orbital inflammatory disease (IOI, orbital pseudotumor).

5. Treatment is with high-dose oral steroids (80–100 mg qd for 1 week, then taper over 6 weeks).

6. Tolosa–Hunt syndrome is a form of IOI involving the superior orbital fissure, optic canal, and cavernous sinus causing decreased vision and painful ophthalmoplegia.

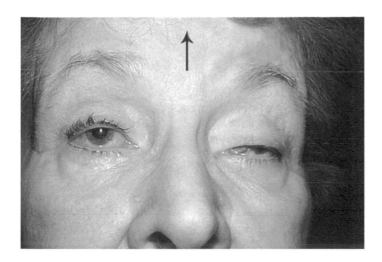

A 66-year-old woman complains of increasing droopiness of her eyelids for 20 years. The image demonstrates her appearance in upgaze.

1. What abnormalities are present?
2. What is the differential diagnosis?

Additional information: eye exam shows BSCVA of 20/40 OU, limited extraocular motility in all direction of gaze (even with doll's head maneuvers), absent Bell's phenomenon, negative forced ductions, and fundus appearance as shown:

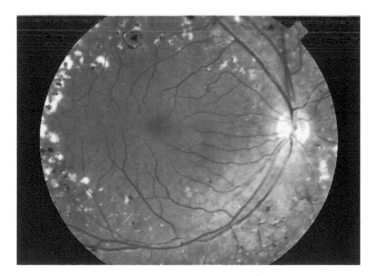

3. What is the diagnosis?
4. What are the features of this condition?
5. Would you perform any testing?

1. The patient has ptosis (left upper eyelid > right upper eyelid) and inability to elevate eyes (limited extraocular motility).

2. MG, CPEO, myotonic dystrophy, vertical gaze palsy, progressive supranuclear palsy, dorsal midbrain syndrome.

3. CPEO, specifically, Kearns–Sayre syndrome (disorder of mitochondrial DNA [gene deletion impairs oxidative phosphorylation]).

4. Ophthalmoplegia, ptosis, retinal pigment degeneration, and cardiac conduction defects (arrhythmias, heart block, cardiomyopathy); also associated with mental retardation, short stature, deafness, ataxia, and elevated cerebrospinal fluid protein.

5. Electrocardiogram to detect cardiac abnormalities (patient should have a cardiology consult). Consider muscle biopsy for abnormal "ragged red" fibers or EMG. Tensilon test, ice pack test, or anti-ACh receptor antibody test can be performed to rule out MG.

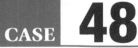
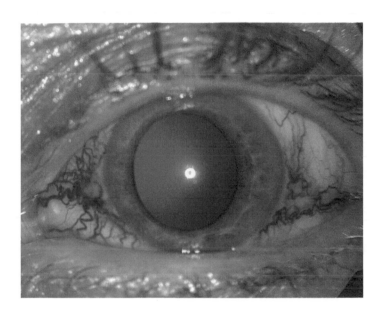

A 62-year-old woman complains that her left eye is red.

1. What notable finding is shown?
2. What is the most likely diagnosis, and what is the differential diagnosis?

Additional information: the patient has a history of head trauma, and an MRI shows a dilated superior ophthalmic vein.

3. What is the diagnosis?
4. What other findings can occur?

1. Prominent, dilated, corkscrew scleral and episcleral vessels.

2. This most likely represents an arteriovenous fistula (carotid-cavernous sinus fistula or dural-sinus fistula). Other possibilities are orbital varix, idiopathic orbital inflammatory disease, iritis, or scleritis.

3. Carotid-cavernous sinus fistula.

4. This is a direct, high-flow AV communication that can cause a variety of other ocular findings including conjunctival injection and chemosis, elevated IOP, proptosis, orbital bruit, dilated tortuous retinal veins, and, less commonly, CN 6 palsy, anterior segment ischemia, blood in Schlemm canal, optic nerve cupping, ischemic maculopathy, and retinal artery occlusion.

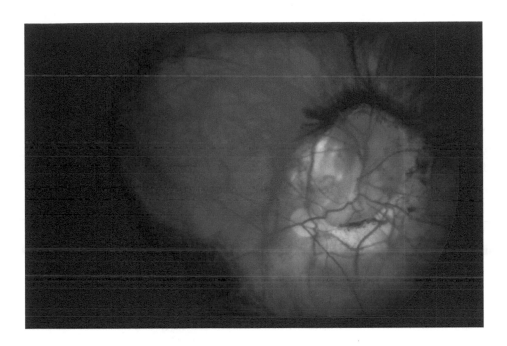

1. What abnormality of the optic nerve is shown?
2. What is the pathophysiology of this disorder?
3. Are there any associations?
4. What is the prognosis?
5. What are other optic nerve dysplasias?

1. Optic nerve coloboma demonstrating a dysplastic nerve head with large abnormal appearing disc elongated inferiorly with an irregular vascular pattern.

2. Incomplete closure of the embryonic fissure results in clefts of ocular structures, usually located inferonasally, and can be unilateral or bilateral.

3. Optic nerve colobomas are associated with other ocular colobomas (ie, eyelid, iris, ciliary body, choroid, retina), and they may also be associated with systemic abnormalities such as congenital heart defects, double aortic arch, coarctation of the aorta, transposition of the great vessels, intracranial carotid anomalies, and basal encephalocele.

4. Optic nerve coloboma causes variable but nonprogressive visual acuity and visual field defects depending on the severity of the nerve involvement, which can be severe (complete chorioretinal coloboma) to mild (slight optic nerve deformity resembling physiologic cupping).

5. Other types of optic nerve dysplasias include hypoplasia, morning glory syndrome (may represent a form of coloboma), optic nerve drusen, optic disc pit, and tilted optic disc.

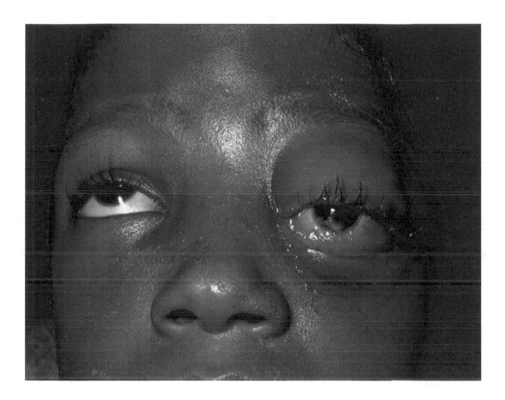

A 56-year-old woman is seen in the emergency department with left eye pain and blurry vision.

1. What is the most likely diagnosis and etiology?
2. How does this condition usually present?
3. What is the treatment?
4. What are the possible complications?

1. Orbital hemorrhage most commonly caused by trauma or complication of ocular surgery (particularly eyelid or orbit) or retrobulbar injection, but can also be due to vascular anomaly (AV malformation, varicosity, lymphangioma) or anticoagulation.

2. Patients have pain and decreased vision, and may have nausea and vomiting. Findings include proptosis, tense orbit with resistance of globe to retropulsion, limited extraocular motility, eyelid edema and ecchymosis, bullous subconjunctival hemorrhage, increased IOP, and there may be a RAPD and optic disc edema.

3. Orbital hemorrhage and compartment syndrome is an ophthalmic emergency requiring immediate lateral canthotomy and cantholysis to prevent blindness. The patient may require management of increased IOP with topical hypotensive medications.

4. Optic neuropathy (from compression or glaucoma) and retinal vascular occlusion.

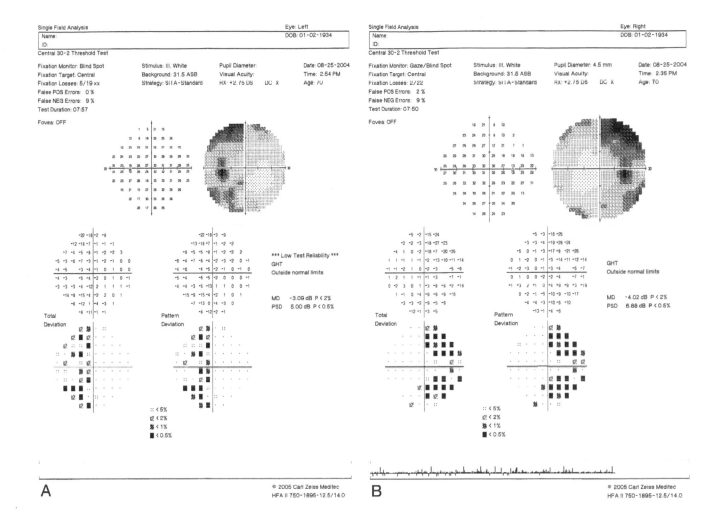

A

B

© 2005 Carl Zeiss Meditec
HFA II 750-1895-12.5/14.0

Λ 43-year-old woman with vague visual complaints and a normal eye exam undergoes visual field testing.

1. What does the visual field demonstrate?
2. Where in the visual pathway is the lesion located?
3. What is the differential diagnosis?
4. What other exam findings may be found in a patient with this field defect?
5. What additional test is needed?

1. Bitemporal hemianopia.

2. Optic chiasm.

3. Most common cause (95%) is mass lesion, usually pituitary tumor causing compression of the optic chiasm. The differential diagnosis includes pituitary adenoma, craniopharyngioma, meningioma, glioma, anterior communicating artery aneurysm, pituitary apoplexy, trauma, sarcoidosis, chiasmal neuritis, ethambutol, tilted optic disc syndrome (field defect does not respect vertical midline).

4. Decreased visual acuity and color vision, RAPD, optic nerve pallor or tilted optic discs.

5. Orbit and brain MRI scan with and without contrast. Head and orbital CT scan in emergencies or suspected pituitary apoplexy.

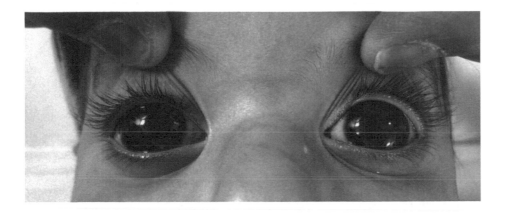

A mother brings in her 5-month-old boy because his eyes have been tearing for a couple of months. On further questioning, she reports no discharge or redness, but he squints and turns away from bright lights. He has no significant past ocular or medical history.

1. What is the differential diagnosis?
2. What exam findings would you look for?

Additional information: retinoscopy shows a refractive error of –1.00 D OU, vision is CSM (central, steady, maintain) OU, anterior segment appearance is demonstrated in the photo, and posterior segment exam reveals a cup-to-disc ratio of 0.5 OU.

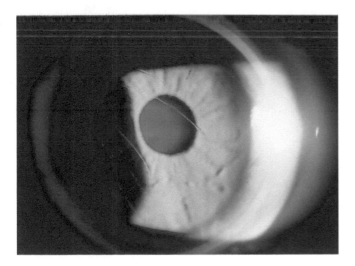

3. What finding is depicted, and what is the diagnosis?
4. What would you tell the mother about the diagnosis?
5. What is the treatment?

1. Possible diagnoses include NLDO, corneal abrasion, foreign body, iritis, and congenital glaucoma.

2. Specific signs to look for on exam include increased lacrimal lake, discharge from lacrimal puncta, corneal staining, foreign body on the ocular surface or tarsal conjunctiva, anterior chamber cell and flare, buphthalmos, myopia, enlarged corneas, increased IOP, and optic disc cupping.

3. Haab striae (breaks in Descemet membrane), which is a sign of congenital glaucoma.

4. Primary congenital glaucoma most often presents in the first year of life, is usually bilateral, and can be primary (developmental abnormality of the angle structures, most commonly due to a mutation in the *CYP1B1* gene). Secondary childhood glaucoma is caused by other ocular anomalies (congenital or acquired) or associated with systemic disease. An examination under anesthesia may be required to check tonometry, corneal diameter, gonioscopy, and ophthalmoscopy.

5. Treatment is surgical. Topical medications are used to control IOP until surgery can be performed: β-blockers are most effective but may cause respiratory distress and bradycardia, carbonic anhydrase inhibitors are less effective and can cause corneal edema, prostaglandin analogs are effective but should be avoided in uveitis, miotics are associated with paradoxical increase in IOP, α-agonists cause respiratory depression (especially brimonidine; associated with infant death, contraindicated in children < 2 years old). Surgical options include goniotomy (children < 1.5 years old with clear cornea) and trabeculotomy (cloudy cornea, children > 1.5 years old, or two failed goniotomies). If these fail, then trabeculectomy with mitomycin C, glaucoma drainage implant, and cycloablation are options. Correction of any refractive error and treatment of amblyopia must also be performed.

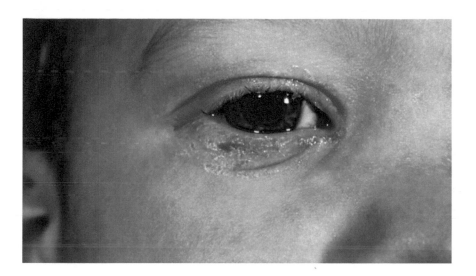

A 6-month-old girl is noted to have a watery eye. The mother says sometimes the lashes are crusty, especially in the inner corner.

1. What additional history would you ask the mother?
2. What other finding would you look for on exam, and what other tests may be helpful?

Additional information: the eye has been watery for 1 month, no redness or discharge has been noted, and there does not seem to be any irritation. The baby has not been treated and has not been sick or around anyone with a cold or eye infection. Palpation of the lacrimal sac produces some scant mucus reflux from the punctum, and dye disappearance test shows delayed clearance of fluorescein from the tear film. The other tests could not be performed.

3. What is the most likely diagnosis and its usual etiology?
4. How common is this condition?
5. How would you treat the baby?

1. Is there any redness, itching, or discharge? How long have the symptoms been present? Has this ever happened before? Has any treatment been initiated? Has the baby recently had a cold or contact with someone with a cold or eye infection? Is there any past medical history?

2. Mucoid reflux with digital pressure over the lacrimal sac and conjunctivitis. Dye disappearance test, Jones I and II tests, and nasolacrimal irrigation.

3. Congenital NLDO, which is usually due to a membrane covering the valve of Hasner. It is bilateral in one-third of cases.

4. Congenital NLDO occurs clinically in approximately 6% of full-term infants and is more common in those with Down syndrome and craniofacial anomalies.

5. Treatment consists of lacrimal sac massage and compresses. Antibiotic drops can be used, especially when there is crusting. If the condition does not resolve spontaneously, then nasolacrimal duct probing should be performed by 13 months of age.

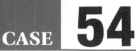
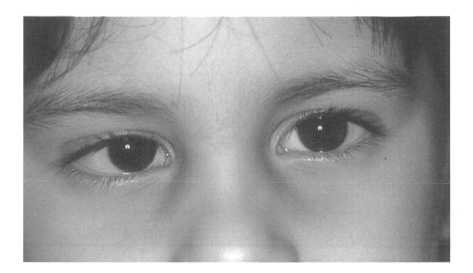

You are asked to see a 3-year-old girl with an eye turn. Apparently the child's eyes have turned inward since she was a baby, but now the mother notices that the left eye also goes up.

1. What is the differential diagnosis?
2. What exam findings would enable you to determine the correct diagnosis?

Additional information: her BCVA is 20/20 OU with +1.00 D OD and +1.50 D OS. The AC/A ratio is normal. The ET is comitant and measures 35 PD at distance and near. She does cross fixate, and there is inferior oblique overaction but no V pattern. There is also no DVD or latent nystagmus present. Worth four dot testing demonstrates suppression OS. There is also a history of strabismus in the father. Anterior and posterior segment exams are normal.

3. What type of ET does this girl have?
4. How would you treat her?
5. If this child also had a DVD, what surgical procedures could be used to correct it?

Additional information: on postoperative day 1 following strabismus surgery, a large XT is noted and there is no adduction of the left eye.

6. What is the diagnosis and treatment?

1. The ET may be congenital, accommodative, nonaccommodative, mixed, or due to Duane syndrome (type 1) or a congenital CN 6 palsy.

2. It is important to know the visual acuity and whether there is any amblyopia or refractive error. What is the AC/A ratio? The ocular motility must be assessed and the deviation measured at distance and near. Is the deviation comitant or incomitant, is there an A or V pattern, and is there any oblique muscle overaction? Does she have a DVD? Is there latent nystagmus? Does she cross fixate? Is there a suppression scotoma?

3. Congenital ET.

4. Rule out an accommodative component by prescribing glasses with the full cycloplegic refraction. Strabismus surgery is performed on either one eye with a medial rectus recession and lateral rectus resection (R&R), or both eyes with bilateral medial rectus recessions. The inferior oblique overaction is also treated surgically with a weakening procedure.

5. Bilateral superior rectus recession, inferior rectus resection, or inferior oblique weakening or anterior transposition.

6. Lost medial rectus muscle after ET repair, which requires return to the operating room to find the muscle and reattach it to the globe, making sure to use locking bites to prevent a slipped muscle.

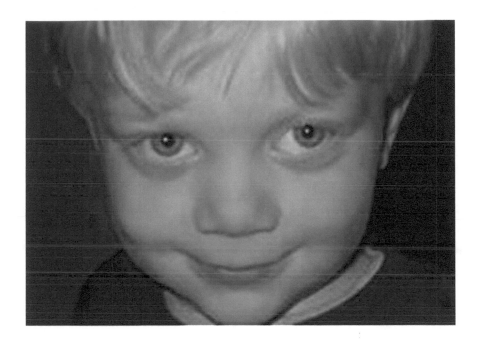

A 3 year old boy is brought to your office because his eyes jiggle. Exam shows horizontal oscillations of the eyes.

1. What is the differential diagnosis?
2. The boy turns his head to the side. If the nystagmus dampens in right gaze, what direction is the boy's head turn?
3. What are the typical features of motor nystagmus?
4. What treatments can be used for congenital nystagmus?
5. What is the triad of findings in spasmus nutans?
6. What is the workup of spasmus nutans?

1. Congenital nystagmus is most commonly afferent (due to sensory deprivation), efferent (motor), latent, or spasmus nutans. It is important to rule out acquired nystagmus.

2. Left head turn to place the eyes in the direction of the null point.

3. The characteristics of motor nystagmus are: usually horizontal in all positions of gaze, increased intensity with fixation, presence of a null point, decreased by convergence, absent during sleep, may have latent component, reversal with horizontal OKN testing, and associated strabismus.

4. Consider base-out prism glasses to stimulate convergence and thereby dampen the nystagmus. If there is a head turn > 50% of the time to keep eyes in null point, then surgical correction with the Kestenbaum procedure can be performed.

5. Fine, rapid, asymmetric eye movements, head nodding, and torticollis.

6. Spasmus nutans is a diagnosis of exclusion, so a careful exam of the pupils (to assess for RAPD) and ON is necessary, and neuroimaging is indicated to rule out a tumor (chiasmal glioma or parasellar tumor, which can produce similar eye movements). Spasmus nutans is benign and disappears by the age of 5 years.

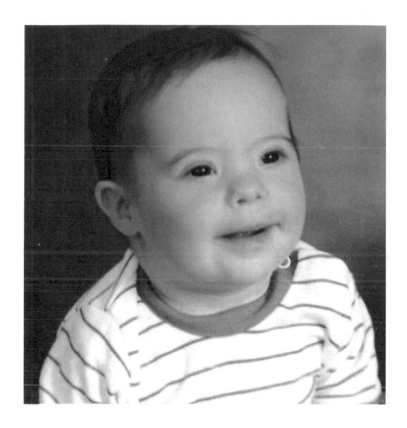

This child's mother brings him in for a routine eye exam. There is no past ocular history.

1. What abnormality does this patient have?
2. What are the associated eye disorders?
3. What are your recommendations for eye care?

1. Down syndrome.

2. Refractive errors (most commonly hyperopia), strabismus, nystagmus, amblyopia, lid abnormalities (epicanthal folds, upward slanting of palpebral fissures, blepharitis, chalazia, NLDO), keratoconus, iris Brushfield spots, cataracts, glaucoma.

3. The patient should have routine eye exams to monitor for associated ocular disorders. Any refractive error should be corrected and amblyopia treatment should be instituted if necessary. Strabismus, blepharitis, keratoconus, cataracts, and glaucoma may also require treatment.

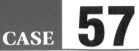
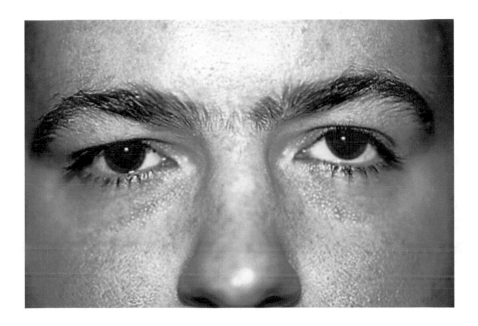

A 16-year-old boy complains of double vision for the last 4 days. He denies any blurry or decreased vision. You notice that he tilts his head to the side, and he says he does this to make the double disappear. On exam, his vision is 20/20 in both eyes, pupillary response is normal, ocular motility shows a left hypertropia. The rest of the exam is normal.

1. What test would you perform to diagnose the problem?

Additional information: he has a left hypertropia that is worse in right gaze and with left head tilt.

2. What is the diagnosis and what other history would be relevant?
3. What head position would the boy have?
4. The patient plays football and says he was stunned after a rough tackle. How would you treat him?

1. Parks–Bielschowsky three-step test. If this shows a SO palsy, then vertical fusion amplitudes would be helpful to distinguish between congenital and other causes.

2. Left SO palsy, which is most commonly congenital or traumatic. This could be a decompensated congenital SO palsy or a traumatic one. It would be helpful to ask about recent illness or trauma. It is also necessary to ask about other neurologic symptoms. Old photographs may be useful to determine whether there was a long-standing head posture.

3. The head is positioned in the direction of action of the weak muscle in order to minimize the diplopia. Therefore, he would have his chin down, face turned to the opposite side, and head tilted to the opposite shoulder.

4. For an isolated palsy, the initial treatment is observation and prism glasses or occlusion of one eye to alleviate the diplopia. If there are other neurologic deficits, then neuroimaging is indicated. The palsy may improve with time. If it does not and is stable for at least 6 months, then muscle surgery can be considered. The Knapp classification is helpful for determining the best procedure. The Harado Ito procedure (lateral transposition of SO tendon) may be used to correct the torsional component.

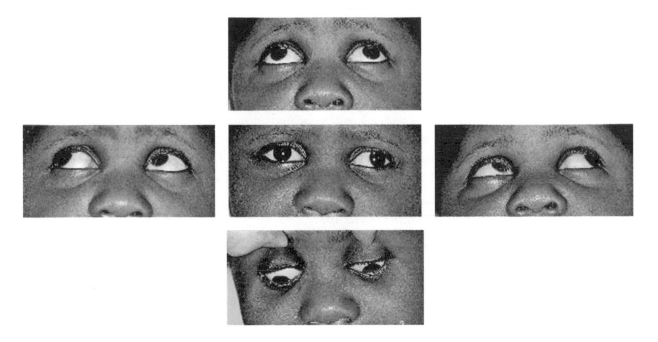

A 6-year-old girl is noted to have an eye turn. Her extraocular motility is demonstrated in the photos.

1. What is the diagnosis?

2. What is the appropriate treatment?

3. Does this child demonstrate oblique muscle overaction?

1. V-pattern XT.

2. Correct any refractive error and treat amblyopia if present. The XT can be treated with overminused spectacles to induce accommodative convergence, fusional convergence training with progressive base-out prism, or prism therapy with base-in prisms. If the ocular misalignment is present > 50% of the time, then surgery is necessary. A prism adaptation test is performed to uncover the full amount of deviation. Surgical correction is performed on either one eye with a lateral rectus recession and medial rectus resection (R&R), or both eyes with bilateral lateral rectus recessions. The V pattern is corrected with horizontal rectus muscle transposition (in the direction of the desired weakening [mnemonic **MALE**: Medial recti moved toward Apex of pattern or Lateral recti moved toward Empty space of pattern]) or with oblique muscle weakening, depending on whether or not there is any oblique overaction.

3. Yes, the photos show bilateral inferior oblique overaction.

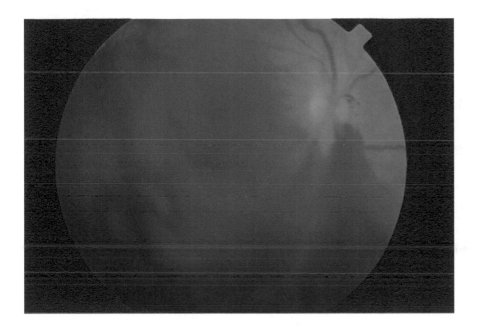

You are called to the emergency room to see a 7-month-old boy because his right eye turns in and he has a funny red reflex. Exam shows poor fixation with the right eye and ability to fix and follow with the left eye. Anterior segment appears normal in both eyes. There is a dim red reflex in the right eye and a normal red reflex in the left eye. Dilated fundus exam shows vitreous hemorrhage in the right eye and intraretinal hemorrhages in both eyes.

1. What is the differential diagnosis?
2. What questions would you ask the parents?

Additional information: the mother says she noticed the eye turn for 1 week. Her pregnancy was uneventful and the birth was uncomplicated. The baby was full term, normal weight, and did not require supplemental oxygen. There is no past medical history and no known trauma.

3. How would you work up and treat this patient?
4. What other injuries are associated with non-accidental trauma?
5. What additional eye findings may be present?
6. What is the visual prognosis?

1. Non-accidental trauma (shaken baby syndrome), accidental head or eye trauma, ROP, Purtscher retinopathy, Terson syndrome, anemia, leukemia, meningitis.

2. How long have the findings been present? What is the birth history (premature, low birth weight, supplemental oxygen)? Is there any other medical history? Is there any history of trauma? How is the baby developing, sleeping, eating? What is the situation at home? Is the baby difficult/crying/colicky?

3. Radiology studies (CT scan and/or plain films) to rule out other traumatic injuries. Report case to child protective services and authorities for suspected non-accidental trauma. The baby must be monitored for amblyopia OD and may require vitrectomy for nonclearing vitreous hemorrhage. He should also have a pediatric consultation and may require treatment of other injuries.

4. Subdural hematoma, subarachnoid hemorrhage, bruises, long bone or rib fractures.

5. In additional to retinal hemorrhages (most common, 80%) and vitreous hemorrhage, other findings include retinal disruption (folds [usually perimacular] and retinoschisis), cotton wool spots, and rarely retinal breaks or detachment.

6. Depends on extent of injury but often poor owing to macular scarring, vitreous hemorrhage, and retinal detachment.

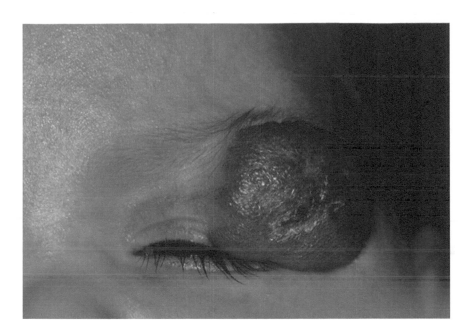

A 9-month-old girl has a puffy, red, blotchy, left upper eyelid that has been present since shortly after birth.

1. What is the diagnosis?
2. What are the potential ocular complications of this lesion?
3. What are the most important parts of the eye exam to check?
4. What are the treatment options?
5. What systemic syndrome is associated with this tumor?

1. Capillary hemangioma, which is the most common benign eyelid tumor in children.

2. Eyelid capillary hemangiomas may cause ptosis or astigmatism resulting in anisometropia, strabismus, or amblyopia.

3. It is important to determine whether the lid lesion is affecting vision. Therefore, it is critical to measure the visual acuity, refractive error, ocular alignment, and motility.

4. Treat any refractive error and amblyopia if present. Most capillary hemangiomas regress by 10 years of age; however, if the tumor is affecting vision, it may require intervention with intralesional (risk of central retinal artery occlusion) or systemic steroids, systemic propranolol, laser photocoagulation, embolization, or excision. Topical timolol may also be effective and is a safer alternative to the aforementioned traditional treatments.

5. Kasabach–Merritt syndrome, which is a consumptive coagulopathy with platelet trapping that causes thrombocytopenia and cardiac failure and has a mortality rate of 30%.

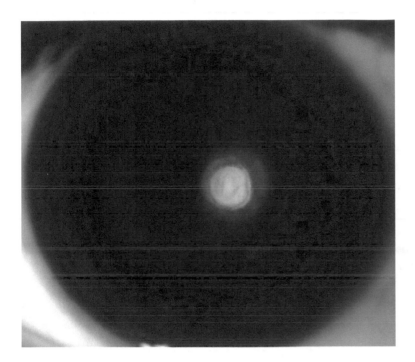

A mother brings her 2-year-old daughter to see you because she notices the girl's pupils look funny in certain lighting conditions. The child has normal vision and ocular motility. Slit lamp exam reveals the abnormality seen in the photo.

1. What is the diagnosis?

2. What is the etiology of bilateral congenital cataracts?

3. What is the treatment?

4. When a patient with the type of cataract shown above undergoes phacoemulsification, there is an increased risk of what complication?

5. What routine step of cataract surgery should not be performed?

1. Posterior polar cataract.

2. Idiopathic, hereditary (usually AD), metabolic, associated with ocular disorder, intrauterine infection (TORCH – Toxoplasma, Other viruses, Rubella, Cytomegalovirus, Herpesvirus), maternal drug ingestion or malnutrition, or trauma.

3. The treatment depends on the size of the cataract and whether it is affecting vision. The critical size for causing vision impairment is ≥ 3 mm. Posterior polar cataracts < 3 mm in diameter should be followed closely for growth and decreased visual acuity. Surgery (cataract extraction and intraocular lens insertion) is performed when the cataract is visually significant.

4. Posterior capsular rupture with possible vitreous loss and/or retained lens material.

5. A posterior capsular defect is often present, so hydrodissection should not be performed since this step can rupture the posterior capsule. Also, polishing/vacuuming the central posterior capsule of residual lens material/plaque should be avoided because even gentle manipulation of this area can cause a break in the posterior capsule. Any remaining opacity can be safely removed with a primary posterior capsulorhexis at the time of surgery or a Nd:YAG laser posterior capsulotomy at a later date.

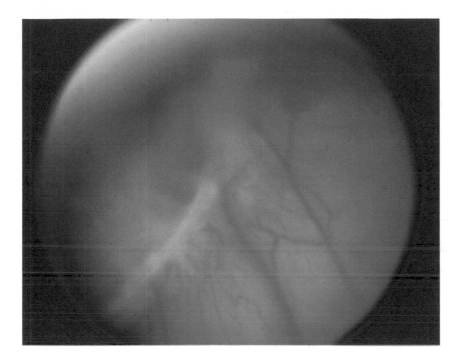

You are called to the neonatal intensive care unit to see a 31-week-old premature infant. The retinal appearance is demonstrated in the photo.

1. What is the diagnosis?
2. What is the classification system of this disorder?
3. What are the risk factors?
4. What is plus disease?
5. When is treatment indicated?

Additional information: retinal exam reveals this baby's disease is zone II, stage 3, without plus disease.

6. How would you treat this infant?
7. What is the prognosis?
8. What are the potential complications?

1. Stage 3 retinopathy of ROP.
2. ROP is classified according to the International Classification of Retinopathy of Prematurity, Third Edition (ICROP3).

   Acute phase ROP: each eye is classified based on the fundus examination.

   Zone: location of disease; 3 retinal zones centered on the optic disc, disease location is based on most posterior lesion.

   > **Zone I:** posterior pole; inner zone corresponding to the area enclosed by a circle around the optic disc with a radius equal to twice the distance from the disc to the macula (60 degree diameter circle centered on the optic disc).

   > **Zone II:** the area between the edge of zone I and a circle centered on the optic disc and tangent to the nasal ora serrata.

   > **Posterior zone II:** the area from the edge of zone I extending 2 disc diameters into zone II.

   > **Zone III:** the remaining crescent of temporal peripheral retina anterior to zone II.

   > **Notch:** = 1-2 clock hour lesion intruding into a more posterior zone (ie, zone II secondary to notch).

   Stage: appearance of acute disease at avascular/vascular junction.

   > **Stage 1:** demarcation line (flat, circumferential, thin, white line between the posterior vascularized and peripheral avascular retina).

   > **Stage 2:** ridge (demarcation line becomes elevated and organized into a pink white ridge, no fibrovascular growth visible).

   > **Stage 3:** extraretinal neovascular proliferation (form the surface of the ridge).

   > **Stage 4:** partial RD; exudative or tractional.

   > > **4A:** fovea attached.

   > > **4B:** fovea detached.

   > **Stage 5:** total RD.

   > > **5A:** optic disc visible; open-funnel detachment.

   > > **5B:** optic disc not visible; closed-funnel detachment.

   > > **5C:** 5B with anterior segment changes (anterior lens displacement, marked anterior chamber shallowing, iridocorneolenticular adhesions, corneal opacification).

   Extent: circumferential involvement in clock hours (30 degree sectors).

   Acute ROP represents a continuous spectrum of vascular changes from normal to plus disease.

   No ROP: incomplete vascularization (specify zone).

   Plus disease: severe vascular dilation and tortuosity in zone I.

   Preplus disease: abnormal vascular dilation and/or tortuosity less severe than plus disease.

   Aggressive ROP (A-ROP; previously termed aggressive-posterior ROP or rush disease): severe, rapidly progressive ROP; also occurs in larger preterm infants and beyond posterior retina.

Late phase ROP

Regression: disease involution and resolution; first signs are vascular (decreased plus disease, vascularization into peripheral avascular retina, tunica vasculosa lentis regression, better pupillary dilation, clearer ocular media, intraretinal hemorrhage resolution) then ROP lesion regresses (thinning and whitening of neovascular tissue); can occur spontaneously or after treatment (laser photocoagulation or anti-VEGF injection), can begin as soon as 1-3 days following anti-VEGF injection, ~7-14 days after laser or spontaneous regression. Complete or incomplete (persistent avascular retina (PAR): note location and extent. After spontaneous regression, PAR usually peripheral; after anti-VEGF treatment, PAR more frequent and extensive.

Reactivation: recurrence of acute disease lesions and vascular changes after regression (incomplete or complete); note stage (ie, reactivated stage 3). Frequency after anti-VEGF rx > spontaneous regression >> laser (very rare). Usually occurs at 37-60 weeks postmenstrual age.

Sequelae: late RD (TRD, RRD, rarely exudative), retinoschisis (after chronic traction from regressed stage 3 ROP), PAR (with increased risk of retinal thinning, holes, lattice-like changes, and late RD), macular abnormalities (small foveal avascular zone, shallow or absent foveal depression), retinal vascular changes (tortuosity, straightening of arcades and macular dragging, falciform retinal fold, abnormal vessel branching, circumferential vascular arcades, telangiectasia, vitreous hemorrhage), secondary angle-closure glaucoma; can also occur in premature infants without acute ROP.

3. Premature birth (<33 weeks' gestation), low birth weight (<1.5 kg), supplemental oxygen (>50 days), and complicated hospital course. The risk of ROP increases exponentially with earlier prematurity (<36 weeks) and lower birth weight (<2 kg) since at 36 weeks the nasal retina is completely vascularized; at 40 weeks, temporal retina is fully vascularized.

4. Plus disease occurs when there are at least two quadrants of shunted blood, which produces engorged, tortuous vessels in the posterior pole, vitreous haze, and iris vascular congestion. This is a poor prognostic sign. A-ROP is plus disease in zone I or posterior zone II, which has a significant risk of rapid progression to stage 5 within a few days.

5. Treatment is indicated for threshold disease (ie, stage 3 + disease with at least 5 contiguous or 8 noncontiguous clock hours of involvement in zone I or II), which represents the level at which 50% will go blind without treatment.

   The ETROP study concluded that ablation of peripheral avascular retina with laser photocoagulation should be performed earlier (ie, type 1 ROP, which is defined as: zone I, any stage of ROP with plus disease; zone I, stage 3 with or without plus disease; zone II, stage 2 or 3 with plus disease). The Cryo-ROP study showed that ablation with cryotherapy for zone I disease was beneficial. The BEAT-ROP study showed that intravitreal injection of bevacizumab 0.625 mg for zone I disease was beneficial, but long-term safety has not been studied. The RAINBOW study evaluated intravitreal ranibizumab 0.1 mg or 0.2 mg versus laser for ROP and showed better treatment success with the 0.2-mg dose. The FIREFLEYE study is evaluating aflibercept for ROP. For stage 4 or greater, pars plana vitrectomy is recommended.

6. This baby does not require treatment. He should have serial retinal exams every 1–2 weeks until the extreme retinal periphery is vascularized, then monthly exams.

7. The prognosis depends on the amount and stage of ROP. Up to 90% of cases resolve spontaneously.

8. High myopia, strabismus, amblyopia, macular dragging, nystagmus, glaucoma, cataracts, keratoconus, band keratopathy, RD, and phthisis bulbi.

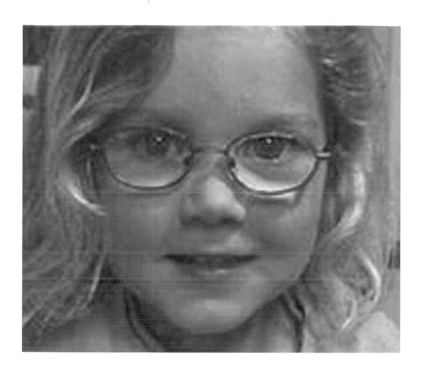

An 8-year-old girl complains of headaches in school. On exam, her uncorrected vision is 20/30 OD and 20/25 OS, manifest refraction of +1.00 D OD and −1.00 D OS yields 20/30 OD and 20/15 OS. Anterior and posterior segment exams are normal.

1. What is the next test you would perform?

Additional information: cycloplegic refraction reveals +4.00 D OD and +1.00 D OS with vision of 20/30 and 20/20, respectively.

2. What is the diagnosis?
3. How would you manage this patient?
4. What are the levels of anisometropia (myopic, hyperopic, and astigmatic) that require correction to prevent possible amblyopia?
5. What are the types of amblyopia?

1. Cycloplegic refraction.

2. Hyperopia and anisometropic amblyopia OD.

3. She should be prescribed the full cycloplegic refraction and patching/penalization therapy started OS for no more than 1 week per year of age before reexamination. This is continued until the vision in the right eye has normalized or stabilized.

   In an older patient who may not tolerate the full prescription, a postcycloplegic refraction pushing plus is necessary and the glasses prescription may need to be increased gradually over time. If the patient is unable to adapt to the degree of anisometropia in the glasses, then consider treatment with a contact lens or laser vision correction OD.

4. Myopic anisometropia ≥3 D, hyperopic anisometropia ≥1 D, and astigmatic anisometropia ≥1.5 D.

5. Strabismic, refractive, and deprivation.

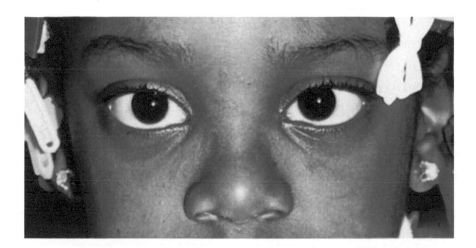

This 7-year-old girl was diagnosed with accommodative ET. Her mother would like a second opinion and brings her to see you.

1.   What are the different types of accommodative ET?
2.   How would you measure her AC/A ratio?

Additional information: her vision is 20/20 OD and 20/40 OS with a refractive error of +4.00 D OD and +5.25 D OS, she has an AC/A ratio of 5:1, and measurement of her ET shows similar amounts of deviation at distance and near.

3.   What type of ET does she have?
4.   How would you treat her?

1. Refractive accommodative (normal AC/A ratio), nonrefractive accommodative (high AC/A ratio), mixed mechanism, and decompensated accommodative.

2. There are two methods for determining the AC/A ratio:

   Heterophoria method: AC/A = IPD + [(N – D)/diopter]

   > IPD = interpupillary distance (cm); N = near deviation; D = distance deviation; diopter = accommodative demand at fixation distance.

   Lens gradient method: AC/A = (WL – NL)/D

   > WL = deviation with lens in front of eye; NL = deviation without lens in front of eye; D = dioptric power of lens used.

3. The high hyperopia, normal AC/A ratio, and similar ET at distance and near indicate that she has a refractive accommodative ET.

4. She should be prescribed the full cycloplegic refraction. The amblyopia OS should be treated with patching or penalization OD for no more than 1 week per year of age before reexamination. Once the vision in the left eye has normalized or stabilized, surgery can be performed for any residual or nonaccommodative component of ET (any deviation > 10 PD that is not eliminated with glasses).

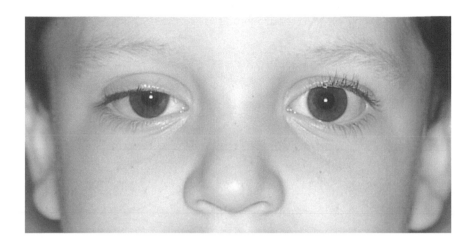

A 4-year-old boy is brought to your office because of a droopy eyelid. His mother states that his right eye has always looked smaller.

1. What are the diagnosis and possible etiologies?
2. What would you look for on exam to determine the etiology?
3. What are the characteristic findings of congenital myogenic ptosis?
4. What is the treatment of congenital myogenic ptosis?
5. What is the prognosis?

1. Congenital ptosis, which can be myogenic (most common), neurogenic (congenital CN 3 palsy or Horner syndrome), or rarely aponeurotic (birth trauma).

2. Visual acuity, levator function, pupil size and response, ocular motility, presence of jaw winking, and iris color.

3. Poor levator function, loss of the lid crease, eyelid lag, sometimes lagophthalmos, and rarely amblyopia.

4. Treat amblyopia if present, then surgical lid repair. For poor levator function, the usual technique is frontalis suspension with silicone rods, fascia lata, or frontalis flap. Maximal levator resection may be useful in some cases.

5. The outcome for congenital ptosis repair is variable and depends on the degree of levator function, poor function being more difficult to treat.

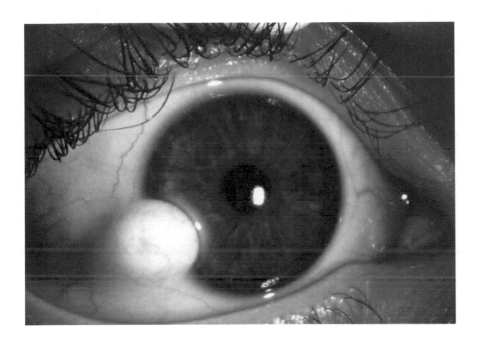

A 23-year-old graduate student says she has a white spot on her eye that she wants removed.

1. What is the diagnosis?

2. What type of tumor is this?

3. Are there any associations?

4. What is the treatment?

1. Limbal dermoid.

2. Choristoma that represents normal tissue in an abnormal location.

3. Limbal dermoids can cause astigmatism and amblyopia. They can be isolated or associated with Goldenhar syndrome (preauricular skin tags, aural fistulas, eyelid coloboma, and vertebral anomalies).

4. Treatment is observation or surgical excision. When excising a dermoid, it is important to pay particular attention to the depth of the keratectomy to avoid penetration of the globe. A variable amount of corneal scarring may remain.

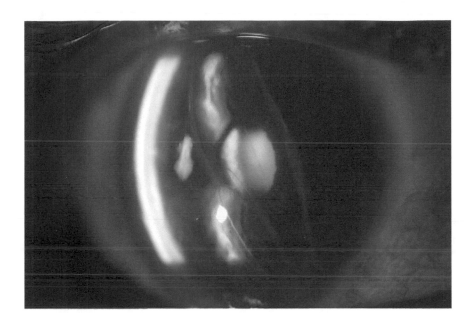

A 51-year-old man complains of a gradual decrease in vision over years. He states that his vision in the left eye has always been worse than in the right eye, and he has worn glasses since childhood for nearsightedness and astigmatism. He has early cataracts that are similar in both eyes with a BCVA of 20/25 OD and 20/80 OS.

1. What anterior segment findings are evident in the photo?
2. What other questions would you ask this patient?

Additional information: his history is negative except for a complicated delivery at birth.

3. What is the corneal diagnosis and etiology?
4. How is this differentiated from congenital glaucoma?
5. What is the differential diagnosis of a congenital cloudy cornea?
6. What are the treatment options for this patient?

1. Corneal scars and cataract.

2. Is there any history of eye trauma or surgery? Is there a family history of eye disease? What is his past medical history including birth history (ie, birth trauma)?

3. Corneal edema and scarring from Descemet membrane tears secondary to birth trauma (ie, forceps injury).

4. The breaks in Descemet membrane from forceps injury are vertical or oblique, whereas those from congenital glaucoma (Haab striae) are oriented horizontally or concentric to the limbus.

5. Mnemonic **STUMPED**: Sclerocornea, Tear in Descemet membrane, Ulcers, Metabolic disease, Peter anomaly, Edema (CHED), Dermoid.

   Other causes include CHSD, rubella, posterior keratoconus, and corneal staphyloma.

6. Corneal transplant with endothelial keratoplasty (DSEK, DSAEK, DMEK, DMAEK) or penetrating keratoplasty for corneal decompensation.

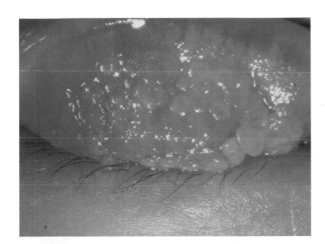

An 11 year old boy says his eyes have been red and itchy for 2 months. He denies any change in vision but occasionally has some discharge. He has tried Visine with minimal relief. His past ocular and medical history are negative.

1. What is the diagnosis?
2. What is the differential diagnosis, and what are the distinguishing findings?

Additional information: anterior segment exam also reveals this finding:

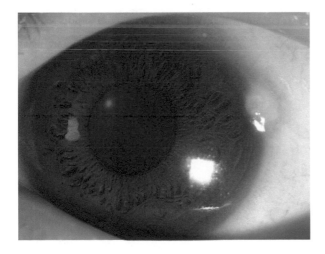

3. What is the finding, and what is the diagnosis?
4. What other characteristic findings may occur?
5. What is the treatment?
6. What are the possible complications?
7. What is the prognosis?

1. Allergic conjunctivitis.

2. Seasonal or perennial allergic conjunctivitis, GPC, VKC, and AKC. GPC, VKC, and AKC are more severe conditions with characteristic findings (ie, large or giant papillae [GPC and VKC], and may have symblepharon [AKC] or keratitis). The age of onset, duration, precipitating factors, associated contact lens wear, and a history of atopy are all helpful in determining the exact diagnosis.

3. The picture shows a Horner–Trantas dot (collection of eosinophils at the limbus). The diagnosis is VKC.

4. Ropy discharge, limbal follicles, and shield ulcer.

5. Chronic therapy with topical steroids and a combination mast cell stabilizer/antihistamine. A steroid with less risk of causing increased IOP and cataract, such as loteprednol, is preferred since patients are young and often require treatment for months or years. The steroids should be tapered slowly and discontinued when possible. Topical cyclosporine may be helpful, as may tacrolimus.

6. Corneal ulceration, scarring, and neovascularization. Steroid treatment can cause cataracts (posterior subcapsular) and increased IOP (and possibly glaucoma).

7. VKC is self-limited. It usually lasts up to 10 years and then resolves. The prognosis is very good if complications do not occur.

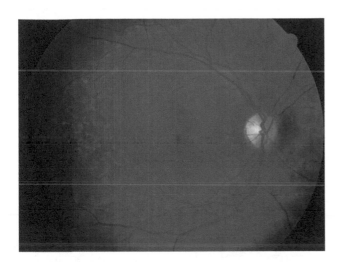

A 20-year-old man presents with progressively decreased vision and similar retinal findings in both eyes.

1. What does the picture show?
2. What is the differential diagnosis?
3. What other test may be useful to determine the correct diagnosis?

Additional information: an FA is performed.

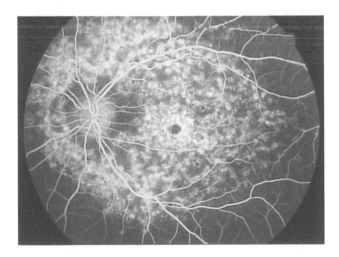

4. What does the FA show, and what is the diagnosis?
5. How would you treat this patient?
6. What would you tell this patient about the genetics of this disease?
7. What is the prognosis?

1. Deep, symmetric, yellow pisciform (fish-tail shaped) flecks (yellow flecks are groups of enlarged RPE cells packed with a granular substance with ultrastructural, autofluorescent, and histochemical properties consistent with lipofuscin) scattered throughout the posterior pole at the level of the RPE. There is also a "bull's eye" atrophic maculopathy with "beaten bronze" appearance.

2. The pisciform lesions with "bull's eye" maculopathy is most consistent with Stargardt disease, but other causes of a bull's eye include pericentral retinitis pigmentosa, cone and cone-rod dystrophy, ARMD, central areolar choroidal dystrophy, chloroquine/hydroxychloroquine retinal toxicity, chronic macular hole, olivopontocerebellar atrophy, and ceroid lipofuscinosis.

3. The FA can highlight the RPE abnormalities of the "bull's eye" maculopathy, but more importantly shows the generalized decreased choroidal fluorescence (dark choroid sign) and a central zone of hyperfluorescence as well as blotchy hyperfluorescent spots that do not correspond to the flecks seen clinically (note: flecks demonstrate early blockage and late hyperfluorescent staining) of Stargardt disease. The flecks appear hyperautofluorescent on fundus autofluorescence imaging due to the excessive lipofuscin deposition; can also show hypoautofluorescence in areas of RPE damage. Optical coherence tomography shows patchy loss of photoreceptor layers corresponding to macular atrophic areas. Color vision is abnormal. Genetic testing with the ABCR400 microarray can find the common ABCA4 polymorphisms with a detection rate of 60%–70%.

4. Dark choroid consistent with Stargardt disease.

5. There is no effective treatment. Vitamin A supplementation should be avoided. Low-vision aids would be beneficial.

6. Stargardt disease has been mapped to a mutation in the *STGD1/ABCA4* gene on chromosome 1p21–p22 in the more common autosomal recessive form. In contrast, the AD form has been mapped to *STGD4* on chromosome 4p and *STGD3/ELOVL4* on chromosome 6q14 encoding a photoreceptor-specific component of a polyunsaturated fatty acid elongation system. Fundus flavimaculatus (no macular dystrophy; occurs in adults) has been mapped to *ABCA4* gene on chromosome 1p21–p13.

7. Stargardt disease carries a poor prognosis with vision deteriorating to 20/200 or worse by the 3rd decade of life. The AD form has a more benign course with milder color and night vision changes, later onset, and less severe clinical course.

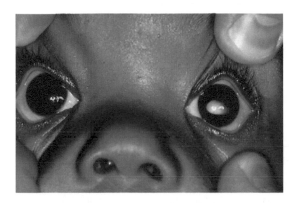

A mother brings her 2-year-old son to see you because she noticed that a recent indoor flash photo showed "red eye" in only one eye. She says it was present in the right eye, but the pupil appeared white in the left eye. On exam, the visual acuity is reduced in the left eye, there is a small esotropia, and leukocoria is present.

1. What is the differential diagnosis?

Additional information: there is no family history of eye disease. The boy has a positive RAPD OS and fundus exam shows the following lesion.

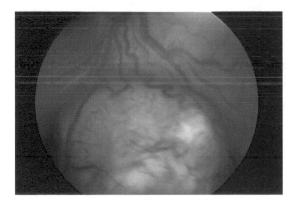

2. What is the diagnosis?
3. How would you work up this child?
4. What are the genetics?
5. What is the chance of a sibling having this disorder?
6. What are the characteristic histopathology findings?

1. The differential diagnosis of leukocoria includes cataract, RB, ROP, and Coats disease. Other etiologies are PHPV, FEVR, toxocariasis, toxoplasmosis, coloboma, myelinated nerve fibers, retinal detachment, and rarer causes such as retinal dysplasia, cyclitic membrane, incontinentia pigmenti, Norrie disease, retinoschisis, and medulloepithelioma.

2. Retinoblastoma.

3. Neuroimaging is performed to diagnose extraocular extension and trilateral RB (bilateral RB with pineal blastoma or parasellar mass). This boy requires an oncology consultation for systemic workup including a bone scan, bone marrow aspirate, and lumbar puncture (cytology).

4. RB has been mapped to chromosome 13q14, and the gene mutation must be present on both chromosomes. RB is 94% sporadic (25% germinal, 75% somatic) and 6% familial (AD with 80% penetrance, therefore only 40% manifest a tumor). Most cases occur sporadically in babies with no family history and are unilateral and unifocal. Bilateral cases are typically familial.

5. If there is one affected child, then the risk of a sibling having RB is 1%. (The one affected child is probably a sporadic case and there is only a 6% chance that it is familial. If it is familial, then the risk of another child having RB is 40%.) If there are two affected children, then the risk of a sibling having RB is 40% (this represents familial cases).

6. There are three characteristic histopathology findings of RB:

   Homer–Wright rosette: appears as nuclei surrounding a tangle of neural filaments without a lumen. This represents low-grade neuroblastic differentiation and can also be found in other types of neuroblastic tumors, such as adrenal neuroblastoma and medulloblastoma.

   Flexner–Wintersteiner rosette: appears as a single row of columnar cells in a ring around a central lumen. This represents early retinal differentiation (ie, attempt of outer photoreceptor production) and is also present in medulloepithelioma.

   Fleurette: appears as a bouquet of neoplastic photoreceptor inner segments. This represents the highest degree of photoreceptor differentiation in RB.

7. What pathologic finding is shown below?

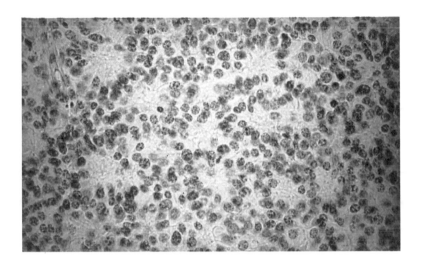

8. What are the treatment options?
9. What is the prognosis?
10. What is the Reese–Ellsworth classification?

7. Homer–Wright rosettes.

8. Treatment modalities include enucleation, cryotherapy, laser photocoagulation, external beam radiation, brachytherapy, intraarterial chemotherapy, and systemic chemotherapy.

   Enucleation is performed on all blind and painful eyes, on the affected eye in most unilateral cases, on the worse eye in most asymmetric cases, and on both eyes in many symmetric cases.

   Photocoagulation/cryotherapy is performed occasionally on eyes with one or a few small tumors that do not involve the ON or macula.

   External beam radiation is performed on salvageable eyes with vitreous seeding or a large tumor, on most eyes with multifocal tumors, and on eyes that have failed photocoagulation therapy.

   Brachytherapy is performed on salvageable eyes with a single medium-sized tumor that does not involve the ON or macula, even with localized vitreous seeding.

   Chemoreduction is when systemic chemotherapy is combined with local therapy and is used in globe salvaging management. Chemotherapy delivered by catheters in the ophthalmic artery or carotid artery have been described.

9. The prognosis is generally good: 90%–95% survival rate and 3% regress spontaneously.

   The prognosis is poor for ON or uveal invasion, extraocular extension, multifocal tumors, or delay in diagnosis. Bilateral RB, degree of necrosis, and calcification do not affect the prognosis. In bilateral cases, the prognosis depends on the status of the tumor in the worse eye.

   RB is fatal within 4 years if left untreated. When metastases occur, they are most commonly to the CNS along the ON, and 50% are to bone.

   About 25%–30% of children with heritable RB may develop a secondary malignancy.

10. The Reese–Ellsworth classification predicts the visual prognosis (not survival) in eyes undergoing radiation treatment. A newer classification system called the ICRB was developed to better predict outcomes:

    Group A (very low risk): small intraretinal tumors (≤3 mm) away from foveola and disc.

    Group B (low risk): tumors > 3 mm, macular or juxtapapillary location, or with subretinal fluid.

    Group C (moderate risk): tumor with focal subretinal or vitreous seeding within 3 mm of tumor.

    Group D (high risk): tumor with diffuse subretinal or vitreous seeding >3 mm from tumor.

    Group E (very high risk): extensive RB occupying > 50% of the globe with or without neovascular glaucoma, hemorrhage, extension of tumor to ON or anterior chamber.

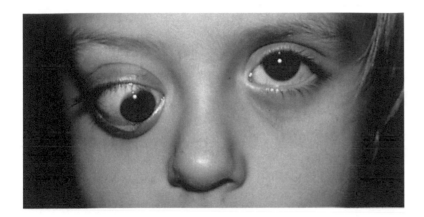

A 7-year-old boy complains of double vision. He has no history of trauma. His past medical and family history are negative.

1. What is the differential diagnosis?
2. What additional history would be helpful?
3. What testing would you perform?

1. The patient's diplopia is due to globe displacement, most likely from orbital cellulitis or an orbital mass. Orbital tumors in children are usually benign (90%). The most common lesions are capillary hemangioma, dermoid cyst, and lymphangioma. Other benign lesions include neurofibroma, meningioma, and inflammatory pseudotumor. The differential diagnosis of malignant tumors includes rhabdomyosarcoma, neuroblastoma, teratoma, optic nerve glioma, histiocytic tumors, granulocytic sarcoma, and Burkitt lymphoma.

2. Is there any pain, redness, or eyelid swelling? Has he had a recent infection or fever? Is there any change in vision? What is the time course of the proptosis?

3. In addition to a comprehensive eye exam with attention to visual acuity, extraocular motility, pupillary reaction, and fundus exam, orbital imaging is necessary.

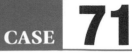
Additional information: a CT scan and biopsy show:

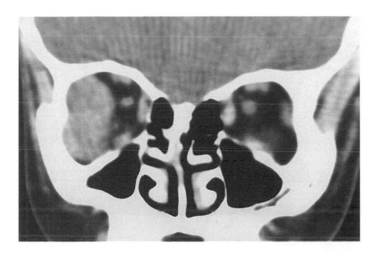

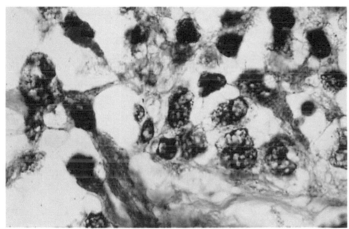

4. What is the diagnosis?
5. What are the histologic types of this tumor and their characteristics?
6. How would you treat this patient?
7. What is the prognosis?

4. Rhabdomyosarcoma.

5. Embryonal is the most common type and usually occurs in children.

   Botryoid is a rare subtype of embryonal, which can occur in the anterior orbit.

   Alveolar is the second most common, has the worst prognosis, is usually found in the inferior orbit, and often arises in the extremities during adolescence.

   Pleomorphic is the least common type, is the most differentiated, has the best prognosis, and usually occurs in adults.

6. He requires emergent diagnostic biopsy with immunohistochemical staining and a pediatric oncology consultation for systemic workup (abdominal and thoracic CT scan, bone marrow biopsy, and lumbar puncture). Treatment is with a combination of surgery, chemotherapy, and radiation depending on the location and extent of the tumor.

7. The prognosis also depends on the type and extent of the malignancy. With chemotherapy and radiation, the 3-year survival rate is 90%. For localized orbital tumors, the survival rate is up to 95%, but decreases to 60% if there is invasion of adjacent structures.

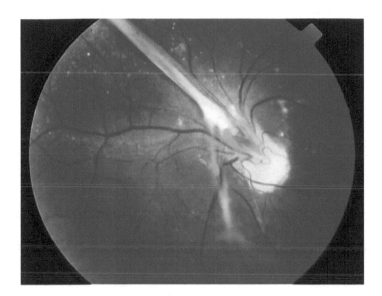

A 9-year-old girl has unilateral decreased vision and photophobia.

1. What does the photo show?
2. What is the differential diagnosis?

Additional information: the patient's family adopted a puppy 1 month ago.

3. What is the most likely diagnosis?
4. What are the clinical presentations of this disease?
5. What is the causative organism and describe its lifecycle?
6. How is this condition treated?

1. Fibrous attachment from granuloma to ON with dragged vessels.

2. The differential diagnosis for temporally dragged disc is toxocariasis, familial exudative vitreoretinopathy, and congenital falciform fold. Other causes of retinal dragging include ROP, incontinential pigmenti, and X-linked retinoschisis, and may also occur in adults with traction retinal detachment, proliferative vitreoretinopathy, and epiretinal membrane.

3. Toxocariasis (ocular larva migrans).

4. Ocular larva migrans has three clinical presentations depending on patient age at time of infection:

    1. *Chronic endophthalmitis (25%)*: 2–9 years of age; granulomatous posterior uveitis with vitreous exudate and cyclitic membrane, which often leads to destruction of the globe.

    2. *Posterior pole granuloma (25%)*: 6–14 years of age; granuloma in macula or peripapillary area, no inflammation, strabismus, nonprogressive.

    3. *Peripheral granuloma (50%)*: 6–40 years of age; granuloma in periphery with fibrotic strand often to disc, strabismus, nonprogressive.

    Other findings: vitreous abscess, dragging of macula temporally owing to peripheral lesion (results in apparent XT), often presents with leukocoria, may have traction RD.

    Rare presentations: pars planitis, ON granuloma, diffuse unilateral subacute neuroretinitis

    Visceral larva migrans: usually in children aged < 3 years; fever, rash, malaise, lymphadenopathy, hepatomegaly, pneumonitis, eosinophilia, meningoencephalitis; no eye involvement.

5. Infection due to the second-stage larval form of the common roundworm *Toxocara canis* or *Toxocara cati*. The nematode lives in dog or cat intestines. The mature adult releases eggs that are passed in the stool. Contact with infected fecal material leads to human infection (more common in children and young adults), but the roundworm cannot sexually mature. Local inflammatory reactions lead to encapsulation of the worm. Seroprevalence is approximately 5% in US population, with higher prevalence in the South. Risk factors include contact with puppies and kittens and eating dirt (pica); older dogs are less likely to cause infection.

6. Antiparasitic therapy with albendazole is unproven. Treatment is largely based on reducing the inflammation using steroids. In the presence of inflammation, dilating drops should also be used. In 25% of cases, vitreoretinal surgery to treat ERM, traction RD, and/or vitreous hemorrhage is required.

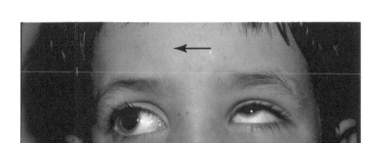

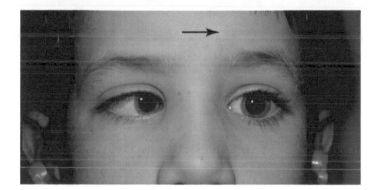

A 10-year-old girl is examined for a new pair of glasses and is noted to have a left head turn.

1. What abnormality does this child have?
2. What additional history and testing would you obtain?

Additional information: the mother reports a normal pregnancy and full-term delivery, and says that her daughter is healthy and takes no medication but that her left eye looks smaller than the right. There is no family history of eye disease, and the only past ocular history is low myopia for which she wears glasses at school. On exam, the BSCVA is 20/20 OU, the eyes appear straight in primary position, extraocular motility is full OD and limited in both abduction and adduction OS as demonstrated in the photos. There is a small left head turn to improve fusion.

3. What is the diagnosis?
4. How is this condition classified?
5. What is the etiology?
6. What other findings occur?
7. What is the treatment?

1. The photos demonstrate limited abduction and adduction OS. There is also narrowing of the left palpebral fissure and elevation of the left eye with attempted adduction, and widening of the left palpebral fissure on attempted abduction.

2. A complete history must be obtained including birth history (ie, prematurity), past ocular history (visual acuity, glasses use, any trauma, surgery, strabismus, patching/penalization), family history of eye disorders, past medical history and medications. A complete eye exam should be performed with attention to visual acuity, refraction, fusion and motility tests (cover-uncover, and alternate cover).

3. Duane retraction syndrome type 3.

4. There are three types (1 > 3 > 2), the left eye is affected more commonly, and 20% are bilateral:

   Type 1: limited abduction, esotropia in primary position

   Type 2: limited adduction, exotropia in primary position

   Type 3: limited abduction and adduction.

5. Congenital agenesis or hypoplasia of the abducens nerve (CN 6) and abnormal innervation of the lateral rectus muscle by a branch of CN 3.

6. In addition to limitations of horizontal motility, cocontraction of the medial and lateral rectus muscles result in globe retraction and narrowing of the palpebral fissure. The palpebral fissure of the affected side narrows on adduction and widens on abduction. Vertical deviations referred to as upshoots and downshoots (leash phenomenon) often occur, and the patient may have a head turn to fuse. Other associated abnormalities are deafness, crocodile tears, syndromes (Goldenhar syndrome, Klippel–Feil syndrome, Wildervanck syndrome, fetal alcohol syndrome, cat eye syndrome), and other findings of prenatal thalidomide exposure.

7. Any refractive error should be corrected and amblyopia should be treated. Otherwise, Duane syndrome usually does not require treatment, but indications for muscle surgery include a deviation in primary position, abnormal head position, or significant upshoot or downshoot.

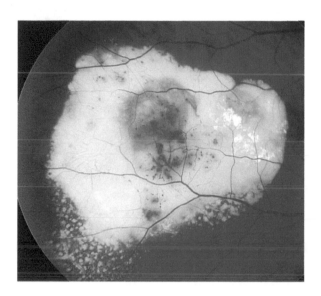

A 6-year-old boy presents with unilateral leukocoria.

1. What findings are evident in the photo?
2. What is the differential diagnosis?

Additional information: the FA shows:

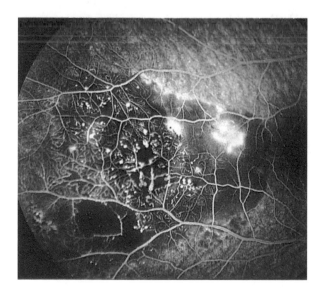

3. Describe the FA findings. What is the diagnosis?
4. What is the staging of this disease?
5. How would you treat this patient?
6. What is the prognosis?

1. Retinal telangiectasia with extensive leaking telangiectatic vessels, massive lipid exudates, and an exudative RD.

2. Coats disease, PHPV, RB, angiomatosis retinae.

3. The FA demonstrates large telangiectatic vessels and numerous leaking aneurysms ("light bulb" dilatations). This is the classic presentation of Coats disease.

4. There are two staging schema for Coats disease:

   Gomez–Morales staging

   Stage I: focal exudates

   Stage II: massive exudation

   Stage III: partial exudative RD

   Stage IV: total RD

   Stage V: complications

   Sigelman staging

   Stage I: only telangiectasia

   Stage II: focal exudates

   Stage III: partial exudative RD

   Stage IV: total RD

   Stage V: complications

   Coats disease represents the severe form of a spectrum of disease. It usually affects males (10:1) < 20 years of age (2/3 before age 10 years) and is unilateral (80%–95%). The milder form is Leber miliary aneurysms, which occurs in older individuals, affects men and women equally, and is usually bilateral.

5. Laser treatment, cryotherapy, and anti-VEGF injections have all been tried.

6. The prognosis depends on the stage of the disease. The older the patient at presentation, the better the prognosis; often the prognosis is poor when presenting before 3 years of age.

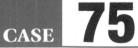
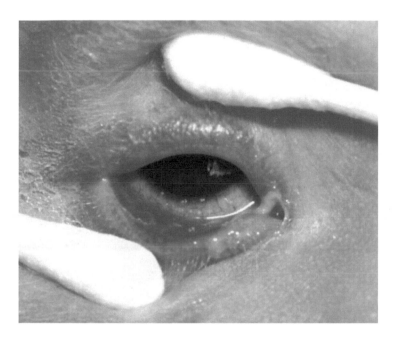

A 6-day-old infant is found to have redness and discharge from both eyes.

1.   What questions would you ask the mother?

2.   What is the diagnosis?

3.   What are the possible etiologies and characteristic features?

Additional information: the mother reports a normal full-term vaginal delivery and no premature rupture of the membranes. She has no history of HSV or Neisseria gonorrhoeae (GC). The infant received topical erythromycin ointment OU at the hospital and has not had any medication since and has no other signs or symptoms of infection. The redness and discharge began 1 day ago, and the discharge is yellow and moderate in quantity.

4.   What is the most likely cause?

5.   How would you work up this infant?

6.   What is the appropriate treatment?

1. It is helpful to know when the redness and discharge began. What is the quantity and quality of the discharge? Does the baby have a fever or any other signs of infection (runny nose, cough, rash, lethargy, emesis, etc.)? Has the baby received any medications? Was the birth vaginal or C-section? Were there any complications? Does the mother have any communicable diseases?

2. Conjunctivitis, specifically ophthalmia neonatorum.

3. *Chemical (silver nitrate 1% solution)*: occurs in first 24 hours with mild clear watery discharge and conjunctival injection, and lasts 24–36 hours.

   Bacterial: *Neisseria gonorrhoeae* occurs on day 3-4, or earlier if premature rupture of membranes, ranging from mild to severe with copious purulent discharge, chemosis, lid edema; may be hemorrhagic, develop corneal ulceration or perforation, or systemic involvement with sepsis, meningitis, arthritis. Other bacteria (*Staphylococci, Streptococci, Haemophilus, Enterococci*) present on day 4-5 with scant to moderate purulent discharge and conjunctival injection.

   Viral (HSV, usually type 2): occurs at 2 weeks with serous discharge, conjunctival injection, keratitis, may have eyelid vesicles.

   Chlamydial (Chlamydia trachomatis neonatal inclusion conjunctivitis): most common, occurs at approximately 1 week with mild to moderate filmy discharge, lid edema, conjunctival papillae (not follicles), may have pseudomembranes; associated with pneumonitis, otitis, nasopharyngitis, gastritis.

4. Bacterial, most likely *Haemophilus influenzae* or *Streptococcus pneumoniae.*

5. Gram stain and culture to determine the organism.

6. Empiric topical antibiotic (bacitracin, erythromycin, or tetracycline ointment) for 7 days; may require systemic antibiotic for extraocular involvement (ie, otitis media).

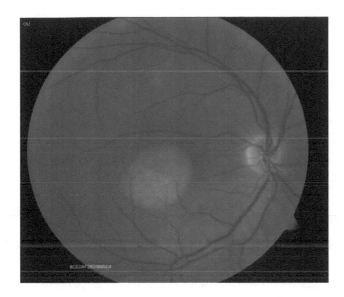

A 26-year-old man has a history of reduced vision.

1. What is the differential diagnosis?
2. What diagnostic tests should you perform?

Additional information: the OCT shows:

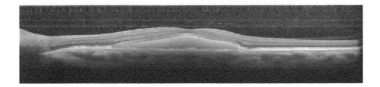

3. What is the diagnosis?
4. What is the etiology?
5. Describe the pathophysiology and stages of this disease.

1. Best disease or vitelliform macular dystrophy (most likely), adult foveomacular vitelliform dystrophy, age-related macular degeneration, North Carolina macular dystrophy, macular coloboma, dominant drusen, central serous chorioretinopathy, solar retinopathy, macular hole, toxoplasmosis, myopic degeneration, old foveal hemorrhage, syphilis, autosomal recessive bestrophinopathy, AD vitreoretinochoroidopathy.

2. Usually diagnosed by clinical examination, but EOG shows an abnormal Arden ratio with normal ERG. OCT nicely demonstrates the vitelliform lesion. FA shows hypofluorescent blockage of the vitelliform lesion. Fundus autofluorescence shows hyperautofluorescence in the early stages and hypoautofluorescence during the atrophic stage. Genetic testing for the *BEST1* gene on the long arm of chromosome 11, which encodes the transmembrane protein bestrophin1.

3. The OCT shows a vitelliform lesion consistent with Best disease.

4. Best disease is a hereditary (AD) macular dystrophy caused by mutations in the *BEST1* gene on chromosome 11q12-q13.1.

5. Primary disturbance of the RPE leading to a buildup of lipofuscin within the RPE and sub-RPE space. In late stage, secondary loss of overlying photoreceptors occurs. There are six stages of Best disease:

   Stage I (Previtelliform): normal or subtle RPE changes, small, round, central yellow spot. Normal vision, FA shows RPE window defects, abnormal EOG.

   Stage II (Vitelliform): age 3–15 years old; well circumscribed, round, classic yellow/orange "egg yolk" or "fried egg" appearance in the fovea, 30% have one or more ectopic locations. Normal vision or mild vision loss (20/20–20/50), FA shows blocking defects.

   Stage III (Pseudohypopyon): age 8–38 years old; layering of lipofuscin (subretinal material breaks through RPE into subretinal space), RPE atrophy. Mild visual loss similar to stage II, FA blocks in area of pseudohypopyon, hyperfluorescent above it.

   Stage IV (Vitelliruptive): breakup of lipofuscin material leads to "scrambled egg" stage with irregular subretinal spots. Vision is mildly decreased from earlier stages (20/20–20/100), FA shows nonhomogeneous blocking and hyperfluorescence.

   Stage V (Atrophic): age > 40 years old; central retinal atrophy with disappearance of lipofuscin material. Vision worse (20/80–20/200).

   Stage VI (Neovascular): Choroidal neovascularization occurs in approximately 20% of patients.

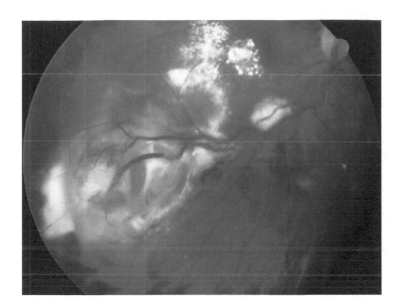

A 21-year-old woman presents with decreased vision in her right eye.

1. What is the finding and what disease is this associated with?

2. Name the six classic phakomatoses, identify the hereditary pattern of each, and describe their characteristic findings.

1. Capillary hemangioma, von Hippel–Lindau disease.

2. Phakomatoses are a group of congenital, mainly heritable, neurocutaneous syndromes with multiple ocular and systemic tumors (hamartomas):

    1. *Angiomatosis retinae (von Hippel–Lindau disease)*: AD with incomplete penetrance (chromosome 3p26-p25 *VHL*).

        Eye findings: retinal angioma (hemangioma or hemangioblastoma; round orange-red mass fed by dilated tortuous retinal artery and drained by engorged vein; may be multifocal as well as bilateral (50%); often in midperiphery, may be near disc; leaks heavily causing serous RD and/or macular edema).

        Systemic findings: 25% of retinal capillary hemangiomas associated with CNS tumor (hemangioblastoma of cerebellum [60%]; pons, medulla, and/or spinal cord is less common); visceral lesions (cysts and tumors of the kidney, pancreas, liver, adrenal glands, including renal cell carcinoma [25%], pheochromocytoma [10%–20%]).

        Von Hippel disease: only ocular involvement.

    2. *Ataxia telangiectasia (Louis–Bar syndrome)*: autosomal recessive (chromosome 11q22 (*ATM*)).

        Eye findings: prominent dilated conjunctival vessels, impaired convergence, nystagmus, oculomotor apraxia.

        Systemic findings: cutaneous telangiectasia in butterfly distribution during the 1st decade of life, mental retardation, cerebellar ataxia (due to cerebellar atrophy), thymic hypoplasia with defective T-cell function and IgA deficiency with increased risk of infections, malignancy (leukemia/lymphoma).

    3. *Encephalotrigeminal angiomatosis (Sturge–Weber syndrome)*: nonhereditary.

        Facial hemangioma: nevus flammeus (port wine stain) limited to first two divisions of CN 5; 5%–10% bilateral.

        Eye findings: dilated tortuous vessels of the conjunctiva and piscleral, congenital or juvenile glaucoma (25% risk, especially if upper lid is involved), heterochromia irides (due to angiomas of iris), angiomas of piscleral and ciliary body, diffuse cavernous choroidal hemangioma ("tomato ketchup" fundus [50%]), peripheral retinal AV malformations, may get RD or severe RPE alterations (pseudo-RP).

        Systemic findings: leptomeningeal vascular malformations (ipsilateral to port wine stain), central calcifications, mental retardation, seizures, pheochromocytoma.

        Klippel–Trénaunay–Weber: variant of Sturge–Weber with cutaneous nevus flammeus, hemangiomas, varicosities, intracranial angiomas, and hemihypertrophy of limbs. Eye findings (uncommon): congenital glaucoma, conjunctival telangiectasia; can have AV malformation similar to Wyburn–Mason.

4. *Neurofibromatosis (NF)*: AD with variable expressivity.

NF-1 (von Recklinghausen syndrome; chromosome 17q11 [neurofibromin]):

Criteria (two or more of the following): Six or more café-au-lait spots >5 mm in diameter in prepubescent or >15 mm in postpubescent individuals, two or more neurofibromas or one plexiform neurofibroma, freckling of intertriginous areas, ON glioma, two or more Lisch nodules, osseous lesion (sphenoid bone dysplasia, thinning of long bone cortex), and first-degree relative with NF-1.

Eye findings: plexiform neurofibroma (plexus of abnormal markedly enlarged nerves; occurs in 25%; 10% involve face, often upper eyelid or orbit; "bag of worms" appearance and S-shaped upper lid; congenital glaucoma in ipsilateral eye in up to 50%), fibroma molluscum, plexiform neurofibroma of conjunctiva, prominent corneal nerves, Lisch nodules (glial/melanocytic iris hamartomas), diffuse uveal thickening due to excess melanocytes and neurons (similar to ocular melanocytosis), ectropion uveae, retinal astrocytic hamartoma (less likely to be calcified than in tuberous sclerosis), increased incidence of myelinated nerve fibers and choroidal nevi (33%), ON glioma (juvenile pilocytic astrocytoma in > 30%; may cause visual loss, hypothalamic dysfunction or hydrocephalus; neuroimaging shows fusiform enlargement of nerve with kinking; if have glioma, 25% have NF), meningioma, orbital plexiform neurofibroma, schwannoma, absence of sphenoid wing (pulsating exophthalmos).

Systemic findings: café-au-lait spots, intertriginous (axillary) freckling, cutaneous peripheral nerve sheath tumors.

NF-2 (chromosome 22q):

Criteria: bilateral cerebellar–pontine angle tumors (acoustic neuromas; cause hearing loss, ataxia, headache); first-degree relative with NF-2 and either a unilateral acoustic neuroma or two of the following: meningioma, schwannoma, neurofibroma, glioma, posterior subcapsular cataract; may have pheochromocytoma and other malignant tumors; no Lisch nodules.

5. *Racemose hemangiomatosis (Wyburn–Mason syndrome)*: nonhereditary.

Eye findings: racemose hemangioma of retina (AV malformation with markedly dilated and tortuous shunt vessels); may have intraocular hemorrhage or glaucoma.

Systemic findings: AV malformations in brain (may cause seizures, paresis, mental changes, visual field defects), orbit and facial bones; may have small facial hemangiomas.

6. *Tuberous sclerosis (Bourneville syndrome)*: AD (chromosomes 9q34 (*TSC1* [hamartin]), 16p13 (*TSC2* [tuberin])) or sporadic.

    Triad of adenoma sebaceum, mental retardation, and epilepsy.

    <u>Eye findings</u>: astrocytic hamartoma of the retina (flat or mulberry shaped with calcifications; usually in posterior pole; consists of nerve fibers and undifferentiated glial cells; occurs in 50%; bilateral in 15%), astrocytic hamartoma of the ON ("giant drusen").

    <u>Systemic findings</u>:

    Cutaneous: facial angiofibroma (adenoma sebaceum; vascularized red papules in butterfly distribution, not present at birth, become visible between ages 2-5 years), ash leaf spots (hypopigmented spots that fluoresce under Wood lamp, considered pathognomonic), shagreen patches (25%; areas of fibromatous infiltration, usually on trunk), periungual fibromas, may have café-au-lait spots.

    CNS: subependymal hamartomas (calcify, forming "brain stones" with root-like appearance; concentrated in periventricular area), mental retardation (60%), seizures (80%), cerebral calcification.

    Other: cardiac rhabdomyoma, spontaneous pneumothorax (from pleural cyst), renal angiomyolipomas, pheochromocytoma.

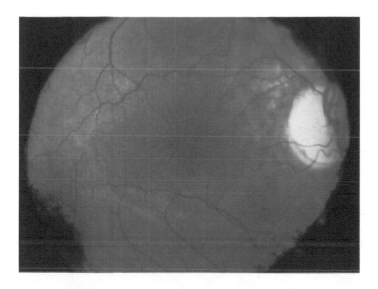

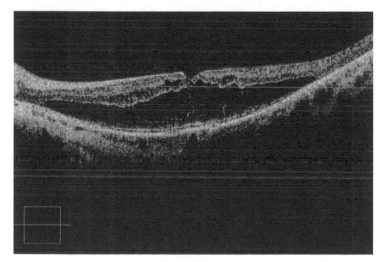

A 9-year-old boy with 20/60 vision is referred for a complete eye exam.

1. Describe the fundus findings and pathology?

2. What is the diagnosis?

3. How is this disorder inherited?

4. What other findings may be present?

5. What are the most common complications?

6. How does the acquired form of this condition differ?

1. Foveal retinoschisis with fine, radiating folds, and spoke wheel–like cysts. OCT demonstrates the splitting of the retina in the macula.

2. Juvenile retinoschisis.

3. X-linked recessive, linked to *RS1*/Retinoschisin gene on chromosome Xp22.13. There are gene therapy trials currently ongoing.

4. Decreased vision, nystagmus, strabismus, vitreous veils, retinal vessels bridging inner and outer layers, peripheral retinoschisis (50%).

5. Vitreous hemorrhage and retinal detachments.

6. Acquired retinoschisis is a senile degenerative process that involves the peripheral retina (often symmetric and bilateral), is usually asymptomatic and nonprogressive affecting the inferotemporal quadrant, but may cause a visual field defect. Outer layer breaks are common, whereas inner layer breaks, vitreous hemorrhage, and retinal detachments are rare.

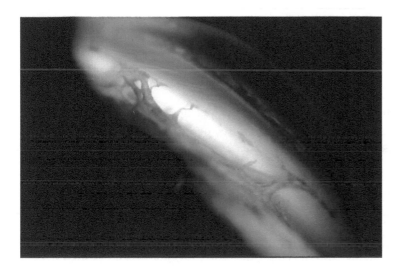

A 16-year-old boy is noted to have a bilateral abnormality on gonioscopy.

1. What is the finding?
2. What other finding may he have?
3. What are the mesodermal dysgenesis syndromes and the findings of each?
4. How is this distinguished from the ICE syndromes?

1. Prominent iris processes.

2. Posterior embryotoxon, which appears as a prominent, white, peripheral corneal line 360 degrees.

3. *Axenfeld anomaly*: posterior embryotoxon (anteriorly displaced Schwalbe line) with iris processes to the scleral spur. Glaucoma develops in 50%.

   Alagille syndrome: Axenfeld plus pigmentary retinopathy, corectopia, esotropia, and systemic abnormalities (absent deep tendon reflexes, abnormal facies, pulmonic valvular stenosis, peripheral arterial stenosis, biliary hypoplasia, and skeletal abnormalities).

   Rieger anomaly: Axenfeld plus iris hypoplasia with holes. Glaucoma develops in 50%.

   Rieger syndrome: Rieger anomaly plus mental retardation and systemic abnormalities (dental, craniofacial, genitourinary, and skeletal).

   Peter anomaly: central corneal leukoma (opacity due to defect in Descemet membrane with absence of endothelium) with iris adhesions, may have cataract and develop glaucoma (50%), and is associated with cardiac, craniofacial, and skeletal abnormalities. It is usually sporadic and bilateral (80%).

4. *Mesodermal dysgenesis*: bilateral, congenital, and hereditary.

   ICE: unilateral, nonhereditary, progressive abnormality of the corneal endothelium that is not associated with any systemic abnormalities. It most commonly affects middle-aged women.

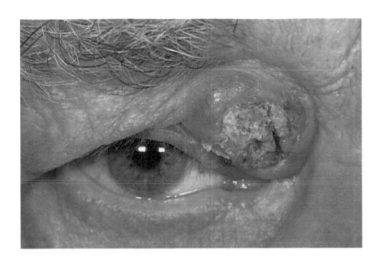

A 65-year-old man notices a red bump on his right upper eyelid that has been enlarging for the past 6 weeks. He initially applied warm compresses once a day without any improvement.

1. What do you think this represents, and what is the differential diagnosis?
2. What would be your next step?

Additional information: the pathology shows:

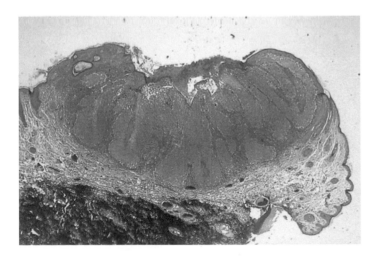

3. What is the diagnosis?
4. How would you treat this patient?
5. How would the treatment differ for sebaceous gland carcinoma?

1. The lesion appears to be a squamous cell carcinoma or keratoacanthoma, but other possibilities are BCC, sebaceous gland carcinoma, inflamed actinic keratosis, tricholemmoma, and Merkel cell tumor.

2. Biopsy.

3. Keratoacanthoma, which is a form of pseudoepitheliomatous hyperplasia and classified as a squamous cell carcinoma.

4. Complete excision of the lesion.

5. Sebaceous gland carcinoma requires wide excision with frozen section and conjunctival map biopsy. Exenteration is performed for orbital extension or pagetoid spread. Radiotherapy is used for palliation.

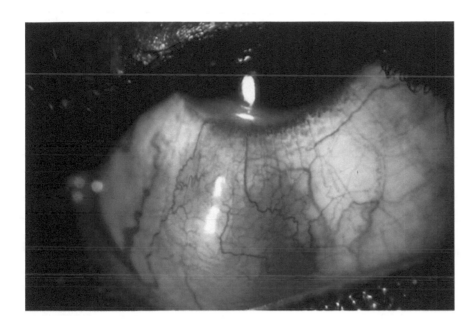

A 26-year-old man complains of a red, painful left eye. He is sensitive to bright light but does not have any change in vision.

1. What is the differential diagnosis?
2. What additional questions would you ask this patient?

Additional information: the patient reports no previous ocular history and does not have any medical problems. Review of systems is negative, and he denies any history of foreign travel or sexually transmitted disease. Exam shows a tender, red, immobile scleral nodule, mild anterior chamber cell and flare, and normal intraocular IOP and fundus.

3. What is the diagnosis?
4. What are the different types of scleritis?
5. What are the possible etiologies?
6. What pharmacologic test can differentiate between scleritis and episcleritis?
7. What disease causes anterior necrotizing scleritis without inflammation (scleromalacia perforans)?
8. What are the signs of posterior scleritis?
9. How would you manage this patient?

1. Episcleritis, scleritis, Tenon cyst, lymphoid lesion, and myositis.

2. Has he had any previous episodes? Does he have any systemic diseases (specifically collagen vascular or autoimmune)? Has he had any eye trauma or surgery? Any recent sinus problems, difficulty in breathing, joint pain, fever or night sweats? Any foreign travel? Does he have a history of a sexually transmitted disease?

3. Nodular anterior scleritis.

4. Anterior (98%) and posterior (2%). Anterior can be diffuse, nodular, or necrotizing with or without inflammation.

5. There is a systemic association in 50% of cases and 30% of cases have a collagen vascular disease (rheumatoid arthritis, ankylosing spondylitis, systemic lupus erythematosus, polyarteritis nodosa, granulomatosis with polyangiitis, or relapsing polychondritis). Other etiologies are herpes zoster, syphilis, tuberculosis, leprosy, gout, porphyria, and idiopathic.

6. Topical phenylephrine 2.5% will blanch the injected area if it is due to episcleritis but will not if it is due to scleritis.

7. Rheumatoid arthritis.

8. Chorioretinal folds, serous retinal detachments, vitritis, optic disc edema, and "T-sign" with thickened sclera on B-scan ultrasound.

9. This patient requires a systemic workup including: CBC with differential, ESR, RF, ANA, ANCA, VDRL or RPR, FTA-ABS or MHA-TP, uric acid, BUN, PPD and controls, and chest X-ray. Treatment is with oral NSAIDs. Systemic steroids, antibiotics, and possibly immunomodulatory therapy may be necessary depending on the underlying etiology.

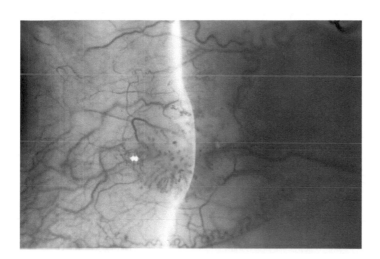

A 55-year-old woman complains of a bump on her eye.

1. What is the differential diagnosis?
2. What would be the next step?

Additional information: the pathology shows:

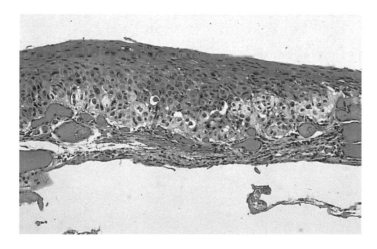

3. What is the diagnosis and why?
4. How would you treat this patient if the pathology had shown squamous cell carcinoma?

1. This conjunctival lesion could be a pinguecula, papilloma, CIN, squamous cell carcinoma, or a lymphoid tumor.

2. Excisional biopsy.

3. CIN, because the atypical cells are confined to the epithelium without penetration of the basement membrane.

4. Wide surgical excision with episclerectomy, corneal epitheliectomy with 100% alcohol, and cryotherapy to the bed of the lesion. Consider topical 5-fluorouracil, topical mitomycin C, or interferon alpha-2b (topical or subconjunctival). Intraocular involvement requires enucleation, and orbital involvement requires exenteration with radiation.

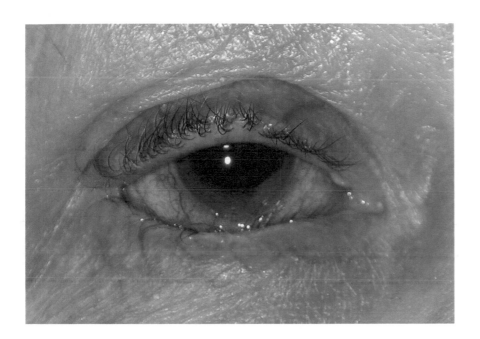

A 62-year-old woman reports that her right eye has been irritated, red, and tearing for months. Artificial tears help briefly but do not really alleviate the scratchy sensation she experiences.

1. What are the diagnosis and possible etiologies?
2. What other history would be helpful?
3. What would you look for on exam to help determine the cause?
4. How would you manage this patient?

1. Entropion. The etiologies include cicatricial, involutional, and spastic.

2. Any previous ocular or periocular trauma, surgery, or disorder?

3. Lid tone (snapback test), lower lid margin position (sagging), and ability to rotate the lower lid by pressing on the inferior tarsal border.

4. The ocular surface must be protected from the inturned lashes with frequent instillation of lubricating drops, gels, and/or ointments. Surgical repair is often necessary and the most appropriate procedure depends on the type of entropion:

    Cicatricial: excision of scar with possible anterior lamellar resection or recession, tarsal fracture, tarsal graft, or conjunctival/mucous membrane grafts. Consider removing lashes.

    Involutional: lid taping, thermal cautery, or Quickert suture; horizontal or vertical lid shortening; and/or lid retractor repair.

    Spastic: lid taping, thermal cautery, Botox injection, Quickert suture, lateral tightening with transconjunctival advancement of lid retractors.

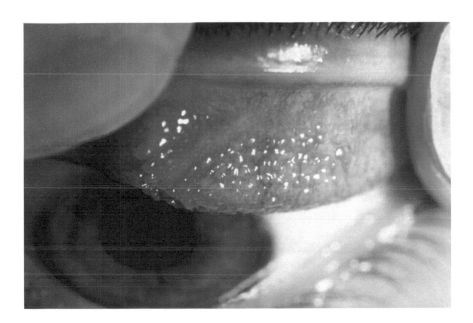

A 38-year-old man complains of intermittent red, irritated eyes for several years. His symptoms are worse in the morning. His past medical history is positive for high cholesterol and moderate obesity.

1. What abnormality is shown?
2. What additional history would be helpful?

Additional information: the patient has no past ocular history, never wore contact lenses, and has no allergies. He denies any difficulty with his vision, can only describe his eye discomfort as "irritating," and sometimes has a little discharge in his eyes when he wakes up. Artificial tears help but only briefly. Exam reveals mild conjunctival injection and a papillary reaction of the superior tarsal conjunctiva. There is no lid margin disease, discharge, or corneal staining. The tear meniscus, tear break-up time, and Schirmer test are normal.

3. What specific finding would you look for on exam?
4. This finding is present, what is the diagnosis?
5. What other conditions are associated with this syndrome?
6. What is the treatment?

1. Superior tarsal conjunctival papillae.

2. Is there any discharge? What is the primary symptom (itching, burning, or foreign body sensation)? Is there any change in vision? Does he wear contact lenses? Does he have any allergies? Does he have sleep apnea? Has he used any treatment?

3. Easily everted upper eyelids.

4. Floppy eyelid syndrome.

5. Obesity, sleep apnea, keratoconus, and eyelid rubbing.

6. Tape, patch, or shield the lids for sleeping. Consider surgery with a horizontal lid-tightening procedure.

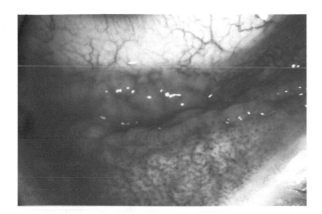

A 24-year-old woman reports red, itchy eyes for the past month. Her primary physician treated her with gentamicin eye drops for 2 weeks with no improvement. She was then given blephamide for 1 week, which helped, but her symptoms recurred when she stopped the drops. She has not used any eye drops for 1 week. She denies any change in vision or mucus discharge.

1. What is the diagnosis?
2. What are the possible etiologies?
3. What are the etiologies of membranous conjunctivitis?
4. What other questions would you ask this patient?
5. What other findings would you look for on exam?

Additional information: she recently had a flareup of sinusitis, but has not had a cold or been around known contacts with an eye infection. She does not wear contact lenses and does not have any known allergies. She denies having a STD. There are no eyelid lesions, subepithelial corneal infiltrates, or preauricular lymphadenopathy.

6. How would you work up this patient?

Additional information: the conjunctival scraping shows:

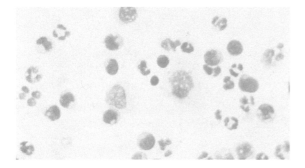

7. What is the diagnosis?
8. What is the organism, and what are the presentations?
9. What is the treatment?

1. Follicular conjunctivitis.

2. Virus (adenovirus, HSV), chlamydia, molluscum, and drug reaction.

3. A true membrane is caused by *Streptococcus*, *Gonococcus*, *Corynebacterium diphtheriae*, Stevens–Johnson syndrome, and chemical burns.

4. Has she had a recent upper respiratory infection or fever? Has she been around anyone with an eye infection? Does she wear contact lenses? Has she ever had a sexually transmitted disease?

5. Preauricular lymphadenopathy, eyelid lesions, pseudomembrane on the inferior tarsal conjunctiva, subconjunctival hemorrhage, subepithelial infiltrates in the cornea.

6. Obtain a conjunctival culture and scraping.

7. Chlamydial conjunctivitis. The scraping shows basophilic cytoplasmic inclusion bodies in epithelial cells.

8. *Chlamydia trachomatis*. Serovars D to K cause inclusion conjunctivitis (TRIC; a chronic follicular conjunctivitis associated with urethritis in 5%), and serovars A to C cause trachoma (bilateral keratoconjunctivitis and the leading cause of preventable blindness in the world from conjunctival/tarsal scarring, entropion, trichiasis, and eventual corneal opacification).

9. Systemic and topical antibiotics with tetracyclines or erythromycins (azithromycin), and also treat all sexual partners.

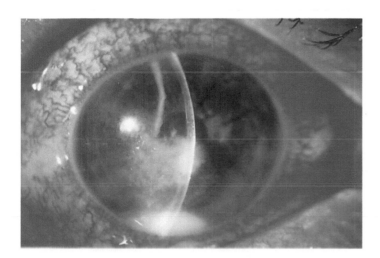

An 18-year-old man complains of a red and painful right eye with blurry vision. It has gotten worse over the past 4 days since he was gardening and thinks he got scratched by a plant branch.

1. What is the most likely diagnosis?
2. How would you manage this patient?
3. What are the indications for a corneal biopsy?

Additional information: KOH prep is positive and a Gram stain of scraping from the ulcer shows the following organism:

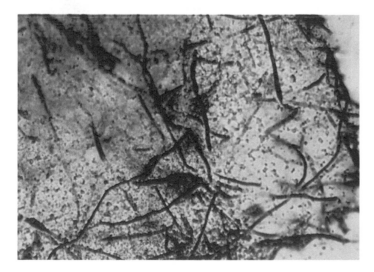

4. What is the diagnosis?
5. What are the characteristic findings of this type of keratitis?
6. What is the treatment?

1. Microbial keratitis, probably fungal or bacterial.

2. Perform corneal cultures and smears of the ulcer and start empiric antibiotic treatment with topical fortified antibiotics (cefazolin and tobramycin) alternating every hour initially, and a cycloplegic drop. Ask the patient about contact lens wear and if he does wear contacts, the lens and case should be cultured as well. This vision-threatening corneal infection initially requires daily follow-up monitoring the vision, IOP, size, depth, and density of the corneal infiltrate, and presence and size of any overlying epithelial defect. Therapy should be adjusted based on the culture and sensitivity results. Confocal microscopy if available is useful for identifying fungi and *Acanthamoeba*.

3. A biopsy should be considered for progressive disease, a culture-negative ulcer, or a deep abscess.

4. Fungal keratitis. The scraping shows branching fungal hyphae of *Fusarium*.

5. Fungal ulcers usually have feathery edges, endothelial plaque, satellite infiltrates, and may penetrate Descemet membrane.

6. Topical antifungal (natamycin, amphotericin B, miconazole, or voriconazole) and cycloplegic drops. Topical natamycin is better for filamentous fungi particularly *Fusarium* (MUTT I). Topical steroids are contraindicated. For severe infection, add systemic antifungal (ketoconazole or amphotericin B). There is no benefit of adding oral voriconazole for severe filamentous fungal ulcers, but consider for *Fusarium* (MUTT II).

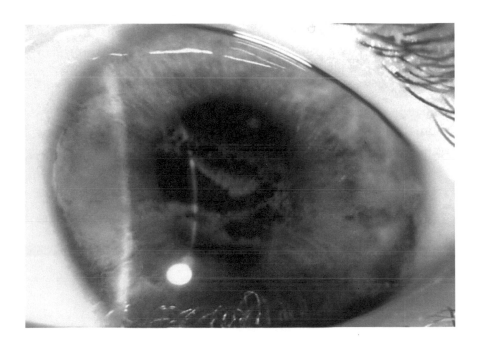

A 46-year-old man has a history of multiple ocular surgeries for glaucoma and cataract. He reports deterioration of his vision in the left eye. He notices a white film on the eye but denies any pain.

1. What is the diagnosis?

2. What is the pathology?

3. With which ocular disease is this most commonly associated?

4. How would you treat this patient?

5. What is the prognosis?

1. Band keratopathy.

2. Band keratopathy consists of calcium deposition in the cornea (epithelial basement membrane, Bowman membrane, and anterior stroma) with destruction of Bowman membrane. It is usually due to chronic ocular inflammation but also some systemic diseases (ie, hypercalcemia, gout).

3. Chronic uveitis (usually juvenile idiopathic arthritis–associated anterior uveitis). It can also occur with interstitial keratitis, phthisis, and trauma.

4. Chelation with topical sodium EDTA. Other options include superficial keratectomy or phototherapeutic keratectomy.

5. The calcium deposits reaccumulate, but EDTA chelation can be repeated.

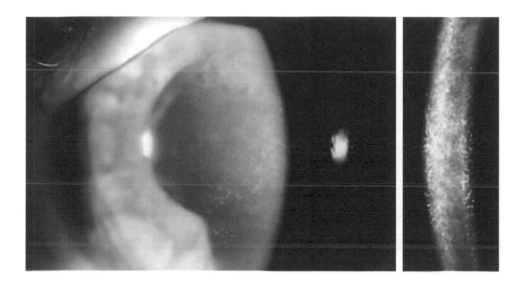

A 54-year-old accountant notices a gradual decrease in vision. She was told of cataracts by her optometrist and referred for a surgical evaluation. She reports increased sensitivity to light and halos around lights, especially at night. Some days the vision is better than others. On exam, her vision with her current glasses is 20/30 OD and 20/40 OS without improvement on pinhole or manifest refraction. She has 1+ nuclear sclerotic cataracts and a normal fundus in both eyes.

1. What other history would be pertinent?
2. What additional tests would help confirm the diagnosis?

Additional information: there is no family history of eye problems. She does notice that her vision is blurrier in the morning and clearer later in the day. Corneal pachymetry is 632 microns OD and 664 microns OS, and endothelial cell counts are decreased OU.

3. What is the diagnosis?
4. What are the treatment options?
5. What are the possible complications of surgery?

1. Is there a family history of eye disease or surgery (ie, corneal transplant)? Does the vision fluctuate throughout the day or with different geographic locations (worse in the morning or in humid environments)?

2. Corneal pachymetry and specular microscopy.

3. Fuchs endothelial dystrophy.

4. Medical treatment consists of hypertonic ointment at bedtime and drops during the day. A course of topical steroids may be helpful. Surgical treatment is corneal transplantation with EK (DSAEK, DMEK).

5. Graft dislocation, graft rejection, graft failure, hemorrhage, infection, and glaucoma.

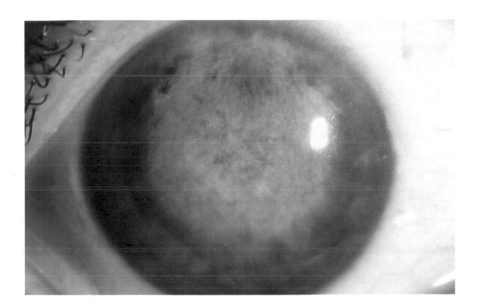

A 42-year-old man has a history of poor vision. The appearance of his right eye is shown.

1. What is the most likely diagnosis?
2. What are the etiologies?
3. What other findings are seen in congenital syphilis?
4. What triad of findings characterizes Cogan syndrome?
5. What is the treatment of active disease?
6. What ocular treatment would you offer this patient?

1. IK.

2. IK is usually infectious. The most common infections are syphilis, HSV, and tuberculosis; also VZV, mumps, rubella, leprosy, and onchocerciasis. Other causes include sarcoidosis and Cogan syndrome.

3. Optic nerve atrophy, salt-and-pepper fundus, deafness, notched teeth, saddle nose, and sabre shins.

4. IK, vertigo, and hearing loss.

5. Topical steroid and cycloplegic drops for the corneal inflammation, and treat the underlying condition.

6. Chronic, inactive IK with corneal scarring can be treated with a lamellar or penetrating keratoplasty.

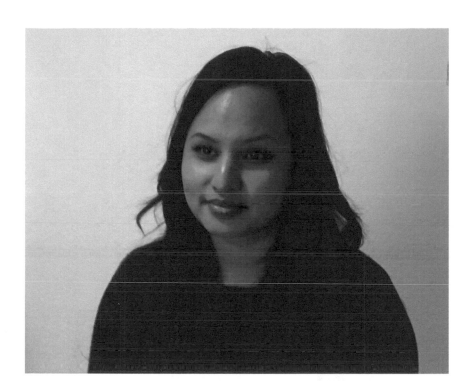

A 26-year-old woman complains of red, irritated eyes for 3 weeks. She wears disposable contact lenses but cannot tolerate them for more than an hour or two. Yesterday she noticed some mucous discharge in the morning. Her primary doctor gave her an antibiotic ointment, which she puts in her eyes twice a day, and she also uses artificial tears once or twice a day. Exam shows scant white mucus strands in the inferior fornix OD and minimal conjunctival injection OU.

1.   What is the differential diagnosis?

Additional information: the eyelids and tear film are normal. There are no conjunctival follicles on the bulbar or inferior palpebral surface, and there is no corneal staining or infiltrate.

2.   What other finding would you look for on exam to make the diagnosis?

1. Blepharoconjunctivitis, acute bacterial conjunctivitis, conjunctivitis due to allergy or toxicity to the antibiotic ointment, GPC, contact lens overwear, or corneal ulcer.

2. Giant papillae on the superior tarsal conjunctiva by everting the upper eyelids.

Additional information: upper eyelid eversion reveals the following:

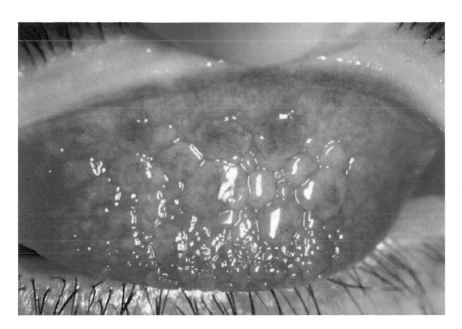

3. What is the diagnosis?

4. How would you treat her?

5. Besides contact lenses, what are other causes of this disorder?

3. GPC.

4. Treatment is to discontinue contact lens wear, use a combination mast cell stabilizer/antihistamine drop, and, depending on the severity, also add a topical steroid. If a steroid is used, the intraocular pressure must be monitored.

5. GPC is mainly associated with contact lens wear, but other causes include a foreign body, exposed suture, or prosthesis.

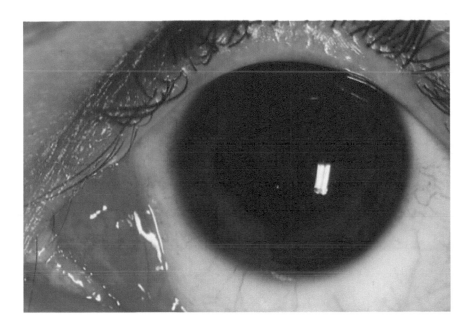

An asymptomatic 57-year-old woman presents for a routine eye exam. Her left eye is shown in the photo.

1. What abnormality is depicted?

2. What is the diagnosis, and what term is used to refer to this type of lesion?

3. What other ocular findings would you specifically look for on exam?

4. How would you work up this patient?

5. What is the treatment?

6. What is the risk of developing systemic lymphoma in patients with an ocular lymphoid lesion?

1. Large, fleshy, salmon-colored conjunctival mass.

2. This is a conjunctival lymphoid tumor and is commonly referred to as a salmon patch.

3. Visual changes, limited ocular motility, proptosis, and lacrimal gland swelling to evaluate for orbital involvement, and lid examination to evaluate for eyelid involvement.

4. The patient requires a medical/oncology consultation and workup to determine whether there is orbital or systemic involvement. Tests include CBC with differential, SPEP, ESR, CT scan (orbital, thoracic, and abdominal), and bone scan.

5. The next step is a biopsy and evaluation of the fresh specimen with immunohistochemical studies to determine the type of lymphoid tumor (benign reactive lymphoid hyperplasia, atypical lymphoid hyperplasia, or lymphoma (50% are MALT), since they cannot be distinguished clinically. Treatment is based on the diagnosis and extent of involvement, and is with external beam radiation, chemotherapy, and surgery.

6. The risk, after 4 years, is 67% for an eyelid lesion, 35% for an orbit lesion, and 20% for a conjunctiva lesion.

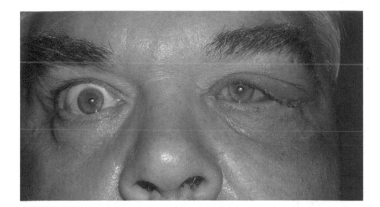

A 48-year-old man reports a tender swollen left upper eyelid and tearing for 8 days. He denies any trauma or change in vision.

1. What is the differential diagnosis?

2. What other questions would you ask him?

Additional information: he does have a fever and reports some discharge from the eye, but there is no diplopia. On exam, he has palpable preauricular lymphadenopathy. His vision is 20/25 OU, pupillary response, extraocular motility, and confrontation visual fields are normal. External exam shows a firm, tender mass of the lateral upper eyelid. Anterior and posterior segment exams are normal. An orbital CT scan shows:

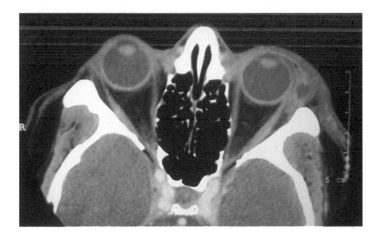

3. What is the diagnosis?

4. What are the possible etiologies?

5. How would you work up this patient?

6. What is the treatment?

7. If this lacrimal gland mass were a neoplasm, what would be the differential diagnosis?

8. What is the treatment of a benign mixed tumor?

1. Preseptal or orbital cellulitis, chalazion, eyelid tumor, dacryoadenitis, or lacrimal gland tumor.

2. Has he had a recent infection or fever, or trauma to the lid? Does he have double vision? Is there any discharge?

3. Acute dacryoadenitis.

4. Infection due to *Staphylococcus*, mumps, EBV VZV, *Neisseria gonorrhoeae*.

5. Obtain a culture and Gram stain of the discharge, CBC with differential, and possibly blood cultures.

6. Treat the underlying infection with the appropriate systemic antimicrobial agents. He may require incision and drainage or excision.

7. Lacrimal gland tumors are lymphoproliferative (50%) or epithelial (50%). Half of the epithelial tumors are pleomorphic adenomas (benign mixed tumors) and half are malignant (adenoid cystic carcinomas and malignant mixed tumors).

8. Complete en bloc excision without biopsy because rupture of the pseudocapsule can result in recurrence and malignant transformation.

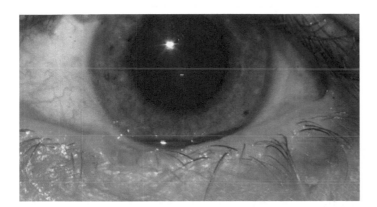

A 78-year-old woman says she scratched her eyelid 3 weeks ago and it bled, but it has not healed yet.

1. What do you suspect this lesion represents?
2. What is the differential diagnosis?

Additional information: a biopsy reveals the following pathology.

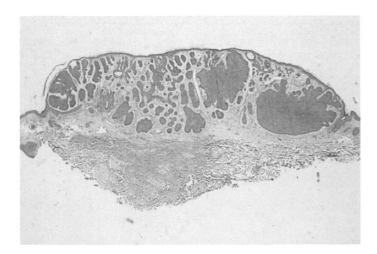

3. What is the diagnosis?
4. What are the characteristic findings of this tumor?
5. What are the characteristic findings of sebaceous gland carcinoma?
6. What is the treatment for BCC?
7. Which location on the eyelids has the worst prognosis?

1. This is suspicious for a skin cancer, most likely BCC because of the ulceration, disruption of normal lid architecture, and loss of eyelashes.

2. Other malignant epithelial tumors of the eyelid are squamous cell carcinoma, keratoacanthoma, and malignant melanoma.

3. BCC.

4. The more common nodular BCC has raised, pearly, nodular borders, and telangiectasia. There may be central ulceration (rodent ulcer) and distortion of the surrounding normal eyelid architecture with scarring and eyelash loss. The morpheaform BCC, which is rarer but more aggressive, appears as a firm, flat plaque with ulceration and indistinct borders that penetrates in to the dermis and can have pagetoid spread.

5. Sebaceous gland carcinoma is highly malignant and appears as a hard, yellow nodule. It can masquerade as chronic unilateral blepharitis or recurrent chalazion with thickened, red lid margin inflammation and loss of lashes.

6. Wide surgical excision with frozen section margin control, Mohs micrographic surgery, and may require cryotherapy or radiation therapy. Canthal tumors require orbital CT scan to assess posterior involvement. Exenteration is performed for orbital extension.

7. Medial canthus because the tumor often extends deeper and can involve the lacrimal drainage system.

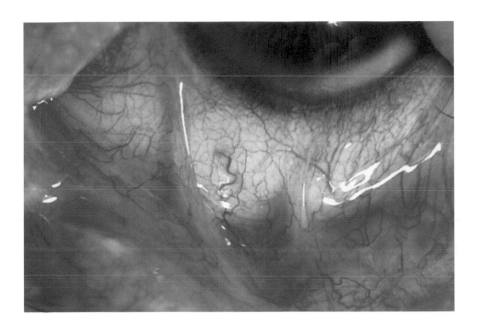

A 71-year-old woman complains of dry eyes for years. The appearance of her ocular surface is seen in the photo.

1. What are the findings and possible etiologies?
2. How do acid and alkali burns differ?
3. What is the acute treatment for chemical burns?
4. How are chemical burns classified?
5. What are the complications of chemical burns?
6. What are the most common causes of SJS?
7. What other questions would you like to ask this patient?

1. Symblepharon, which can be caused by chemical burn, SJS, OCP, trachoma, herpes zoster, atopic keratoconjunctivitis, scleroderma, graft versus host disease.

2. Acid tends to cause less severe injury than alkali. Acid denatures and precipitates proteins, which form a barrier to further penetration. Alkali denatures but does not precipitate proteins, and also saponifies fats (disrupts lipid membranes), causing deeper penetration into the ocular tissues.

3. Immediate, copious irrigation while checking pH level until neutralized (minimum of 15 minutes with at least 1 L of normal or buffered saline, balanced salt solution, or lactated Ringer solution), débridement (any necrotic conjunctiva and particulate matter). Then frequent lubrication with preservative-free artificial tears and ointment, topical antibiotic and cycloplegic. For grades II-IV, add topical (10%) and oral sodium ascorbate (aids collagen synthesis and scavenges superoxide radicals), oral doxycycline (collagenase inhibitor; *note*, acetylcysteine and EDTA are not effective), and topical steroids (for first 5–10 days only to reduce corneal and intraocular inflammation and help prevent symblepharon, but can enhance collagenase-induced corneal melting, which often begins 1–2 weeks after injury; change to medroxyprogesterone if steroids needed after 10–14 days). May require control of elevated IOP, bandage contact lens, or tarsorrhaphy. Symblepharon lysis is performed with a glass rod.

4. *Roper–Hall classification*: based on degree of corneal damage and limbal ischemia; helpful for determining prognosis:

    Grade I: corneal epithelial damage, no ischemia

    Grade II: mild stromal haze but iris details visible, ischemia < 1/3 of limbus

    Grade III: total corneal epithelial loss, stromal haze, iris details obscured, ischemia 1/3 to 1/2 of limbus

    Grade IV: total ocular surface epithelial loss, opaque cornea, ischemia > 1/2 of limbus

    McCulley classification: based on clinical course; helpful for guiding treatment:

    Immediate phase: emergency intervention

    Acute phase (0–7 days): monitor reepithelialization, inflammation, IOP

    Early reparative phase (7–21 days): support corneal healing and limit ulceration

    Late reparative phase (21 days to several months): consider surgery to stabilize ocular surface

5. Dry eye, symblepharon, entropion, trichiasis, anterior segment ischemia, cataract, glaucoma, uveitis, persistent epithelial defects, neurotrophic keratitis, corneal ulceration, scarring, neovascularization, and perforation.

6. SJS is usually drug-induced (sulfonamides, penicillin, aspirin, barbiturates, isoniazid, phenytoin) or infectious (HSV, *Mycoplasma*, adenovirus, *Streptococcus*).

7. What is the past medical and ocular history? Is there any previous eye surgery, injury, or infection? Any severe reactions to medications? Does she have any unusual skin lesions or difficulty swallowing or breathing?

Additional information: she has hypertension, which is controlled on medication. She has never been hospitalized and denies any drug allergies or reactions. Review of systems does reveal dysphagia. Past ocular history is negative except for cataract surgery OS 10 years ago. Since then, her dry eye has gotten worse.

8. What is the diagnosis?

9. What would a conjunctival biopsy show?

10. What is the treatment?

11. What is the prognosis?

8. OCP.

9. Immunoglobulin and complement deposition in the basement membrane.

10. Treatment is with lubrication and systemic steroids or immunomodulatory therapy (ie, dapsone, cyclophosphamide). Patients may require surgery for entropion, trichiasis, symblepharon, ankyloblepharon, and corneal scarring.

11. OCP is a chronic, progressive disease. Surgery can cause exacerbations and should be used with caution. Penetrating keratoplasty has a poor success rate, and keratoprosthesis also has limited success, but is used in end-stage disease.

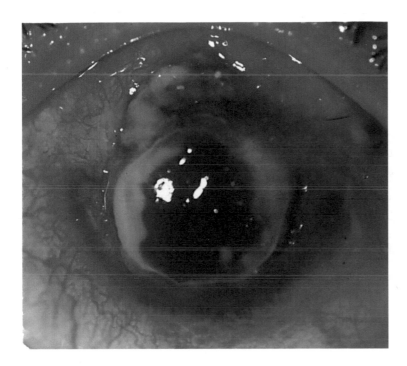

A 56-year-old woman complains of a red painful right eye and blurry vision for several weeks. On exam, there is moderate ciliary injection, peripheral thinning of the cornea, and a mild anterior chamber reaction.

1. What is the differential diagnosis of peripheral corneal thinning?
2. What findings help distinguish Mooren ulcer from Terrien marginal degeneration?
3. What additional history would you like from this patient?

Additional information: further history is unremarkable. The patient does not have blepharitis.

4. How would you work up this patient?
5. The C-ANCA is positive. What is the diagnosis and treatment?

1. Mooren ulcer, marginal keratolysis, staphylococcal marginal keratitis, Terrien marginal degeneration.

2. *Mooren ulcer* is painful and has an undermined leading edge with an overhanging margin, absent epithelium in active areas, and may have conjunctival injection.

   Terrien marginal degeneration is bilateral, painless, and has a leading edge of lipid, steep central edge, sloping peripheral edge, intact epithelium, and superficial vascularization.

3. Does she have any past ocular or medical history? Has she had any previous similar episodes? If she does not have any medical problems, then a careful review of systems should be obtained with attention to autoimmune and collagen vascular disease symptoms.

4. Mooren ulcer is a diagnosis of exclusion whereas marginal keratolysis is due to systemic disease, so it is necessary to order the following lab tests: CBC with differential, ESR, RF, ANA, ANCA, BUN, creatinine, and urinalysis. If infection is suspected, then culture and smears should be obtained.

5. Granulomatosis with polyangiitis, which requires systemic steroids and immunomodulatory therapy (cyclophosphamide). The eye should be treated with lubrication, punctal occlusion, and possibly tarsorrhaphy to heal the epithelium and prevent further corneal melting. Topical cyclosporine, acetylcysteine, and conjunctival recession or resection may be helpful. Tectonic or penetrating keratoplasty may be required for significant thinning.

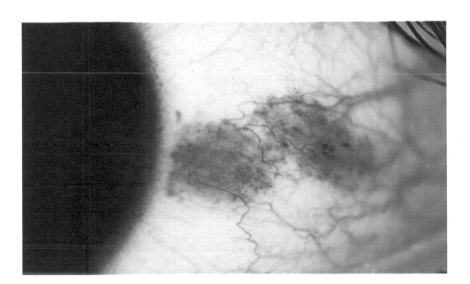

A 44-year-old Caucasian man who has not had an eye exam in 10 years says that he is having more difficulty reading. His eye exam is normal except for the lesion shown above.

1. What are the most likely diagnoses?
2. What are the characteristics of each?
3. What other history would be relevant?

Additional information: he has not noticed it before and has no history or family history of skin cancer.

4. What is the indication for biopsy of PAM?
5. A biopsy confirms the diagnosis of PAM with atypia. What is the treatment and prognosis?

1. This pigmented lesion is probably a conjunctival nevus or PAM; malignant melanoma is less likely.

2, *Nevus*: a discrete, elevated, variably pigmented lesion that contains cysts. It may enlarge during puberty and is rarely malignant.

   PAM: a patchy, diffuse, flat lesion with indistinct margins that does not contain cysts. It may grow (nodular thickening) and involve the cornea.

   Malignant melanoma: a nodular, variably pigmented lesion with blood vessels that does not contain cysts. It may arise from PAM (70%), a preexisting nevus (20%), or de novo (10%).

3. Has he noticed the pigmentation and if so, for how long? Has it changed in color or size? Does he have a history of skin cancer, specifically melanoma?

4. Nodular thickening is the indication for excisional biopsy.

5. PAM with nodular thickening is treated with excisional biopsy and cryotherapy. Recurrence can be treated with topical interferon alpha-2b or mitomycin C. Complete excision is required for malignancy.

   PAM has a low risk for progression to melanoma: PAM without or with mild atypia has no risk, and PAM with severe atypia has a 13% risk of malignant transformation. The greater the extent of the lesion in clock hours, the greater the risk.

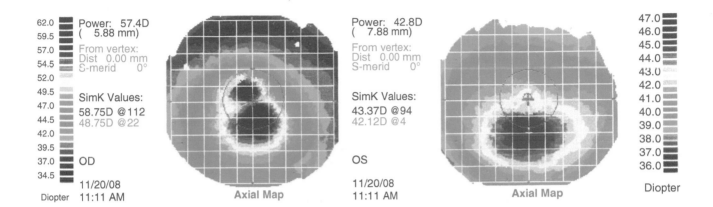

62.0	Power: 57.4D (5.88 mm)	Power: 42.8D (7.88 mm)	47.0
59.5			46.0
57.0	From vertex:	From vertex:	45.0
54.5	Dist 0.00 mm	Dist 0.00 mm	44.0
52.0	S-merid 0°	S-merid 0°	43.0
49.5			42.0
47.0	SimK Values:	SimK Values:	41.0
44.5	58.75D @112	43.37D @94	40.0
42.0	48.75D @22	42.12D @4	39.0
39.5			38.0
37.0	OD	OS	37.0
34.5			36.0
Diopter	11/20/08 11:11 AM Axial Map	11/20/08 11:11 AM Axial Map	Diopter

A 28-year-old man with myopia and astigmatism is interested in LASIK. He does not wear contact lenses. His corneal topography is shown.

1. What is the diagnosis?

2. What is the pathology?

3. Are there any associations?

4. What signs would you look for on exam?

5. How is this condition diagnosed with corneal topography (CVK)?

6. What other conditions may have a similar appearance on CVK?

7. What is the prognosis, and what are the treatment options?

8. How is hydrops treated?

1. KC.

2. KC is a bilateral, asymmetric, noninflammatory, cone-shaped deformity of the cornea due to progressive central or paracentral stromal thinning with breaks in Bowman membrane and superficial scarring. Hydrops is acute corneal edema due to a break in Descemet membrane.

3. KC is typically associated with eye rubbing, Down syndrome, and connective tissue disease. Ocular associations include retinitis pigmentosa, AKC, VKC, Leber congenital amaurosis, floppy eyelid syndrome, CHED, and PPCD.

4. Irregular astigmatism (decreased visual acuity, scissors reflex on retinoscopy, steep keratometry with irregular mires, abnormal corneal topography), apical corneal thinning and scarring, Fleischer ring (epithelial iron deposition around base of cone), Vogt striae (deep, stromal, vertical stress lines at apex of cone), prominent corneal nerves, Munson's sign (protrusion of lower lid with downgaze), Charleux sign (oil-droplet reflex on ophthalmoscopy), and Rizzuti's sign (triangle of light on iris from penlight beam focused by cone) may have hydrops (opaque edematous cornea, ciliary injection, and anterior chamber cells and flare).

5. Characteristic pattern of irregular astigmatism: central or inferior steepening in KC, and similar pattern or asymmetric skewed bow-tie pattern in forme fruste or KC suspects. Most CVK devices contain KC analysis software.

   Three specific parameters can be used to aid in the diagnosis:

   1. Central corneal power > 47.2 D.

   2. Difference in corneal power between fellow eyes > 0.92 D.

   3. I-S value (difference between average inferior and superior corneal powers 3 mm from the center of the cornea): > 1.4 D.

6. Contact lens–induced corneal warpage, keratectasia (after laser vision correction), and pellucid marginal degeneration.

7. The natural history of KC is variable progression with eventual stabilization as the cornea stiffens with age. Depending on the severity, glasses or rigid gas permeable contact lenses, CXL (stiffens cornea), intracorneal ring segments (Intacs), and penetrating keratoplasty. LASIK is contraindicated. CXL should be performed as early as possible to reduce or halt progression with stabilization and often improvement in corneal topography.

8. Treatment for hydrops is supportive with topical steroids, cycloplegic, and bandage contact lens.

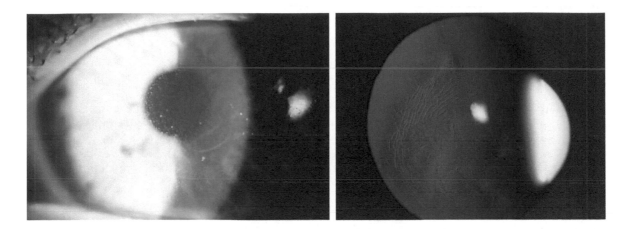

A 36-year-old woman comes in for a routine exam. The appearance of her corneas is shown.

1. What is the diagnosis?

2. What is the pattern of inheritance?

3. What other anterior corneal dystrophies may have a similar appearance with tiny dots or subepithelial scarring?

4. What is the pathology of each?

5. What are the possible sequelae of this patient's disorder?

6. What is the treatment?

1. EBMD; anterior ABMD, MDF dystrophy, Cogan microcystic epithelial dystrophy), the most common anterior corneal dystrophy.

2. Autosomal dominant in isolated familial cases, but the majority is degenerative.

3. Meesmann dystrophy, Reis–Bucklers dystrophy, and Thiel–Behnke dystrophy.

4. *EBMD*: abnormal epithelial adhesion causes intraepithelial and subepithelial basement membrane reduplication with intraepithelial microcysts (dots) and subepithelial ridges and lines (map-like and fingerprint-like).

   Meesmann dystrophy: epithelial cells contain PAS-positive material (peculiar substance), which appear as microcystic dot-like blebs.

   Reis–Bucklers dystrophy: absence of Bowman layer and replacement by granular irregular deposits extending in to stroma, which appear as irregular, diffuse, geographic gray-white subepithelial opacities.

   Thiel–Behnke dystrophy: replacement of Bowman layer by fibrocellular material in a pathognomonic wavy "sawtooth" pattern; curly fibers on electron microscopy. Flecks and irregular opacities progress to reticular or honeycomb pattern.

5. Recurrent erosions (10%) or decreased vision (from subepithelial scarring).

6. Asymptomatic patients require no treatment.

   Erosions are treated with lubrication and hypertonic saline (Muro 128 5% ointment at bedtime for up to 1 year or longer) after the epithelial defect heals. For recurrences, consider a bandage contact lens, epithelial débridement, anterior stromal puncture, or PTK. Also, consider treatment with MMP-9 inhibitors (oral doxycycline and topical steroids).

   Subepithelial scarring causing decreased vision or monocular diplopia is treated with débridement.

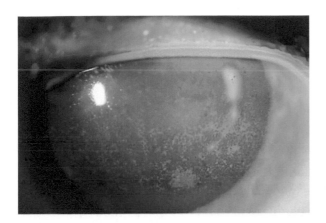

A 32-year-old woman reports a painful eye for 2 weeks and blurry vision. Past ocular history is notable for myopia and contact lens wear. She has never had a problem with contact lenses before and stopped wearing the lenses when the irritation started. Her past medical and ocular histories are negative. She has been using Viroptic for the last 12 days, but her vision has gotten worse and she is very sensitive to light. Examination shows minimal conjunctival injection, paracentral anterior corneal haze, and punctate corneal staining.

1. What is the differential diagnosis?
2. What other questions would you ask this patient?

Additional information: the patient follows a good lens care regimen. She does hot tub with her lenses, but denies any trauma or previous episodes or infections. She is told to stop the Viroptic, refrain from wearing her lenses, and use nonpreserved lubricating drops every 2 hours. She returns 1 week later, and on exam her visual acuity is 20/20 OD and 20/50 OS; there is moderate conjunctival injection, a central corneal infiltrate with mild edema and no epithelial defect, and 1+ anterior chamber cells. The appearance of the corneal infiltrate is shown:

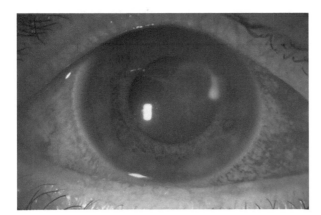

3. What is the diagnosis?
4. What stains and culture media are used to identify this organism?
5. What is the appropriate management of this patient?
6. The patient requires a corneal transplant; what is the prognosis?

1. HSV keratitis, Viroptic toxicity, *Acanthamoeba* keratitis.

2. What is her lens care regimen? Does she use homemade solutions? Any recent swimming or hot tubbing with the contacts? Any recent trauma to the eye? Has she ever had a similar episode or eye infection in the past?

3. *Acanthamoeba* keratitis.

4. Stains: Giemsa and Calcofluor white.

   Culture media: nonnutrient agar with *Escherichia coli* overgrowth.

5. Topical treatment with a combination of antibacterial, antifungal, and antiparasitic agents for months: neomycin or paromomycin; miconazole or clotrimazole (and oral voriconazole, ketoconazole or itraconazole); Brolene or hexamidine; and Baquacil or chlorhexidine. A topical cycloplegic drop should also be prescribed, and epithelial débridement should be considered. Topical steroids are controversial, but consider for inflammation after the infection has been controlled or if severe necrotizing keratitis develops. Oral NSAIDs for pain.

6. There is a 30% recurrence rate after penetrating keratoplasty.

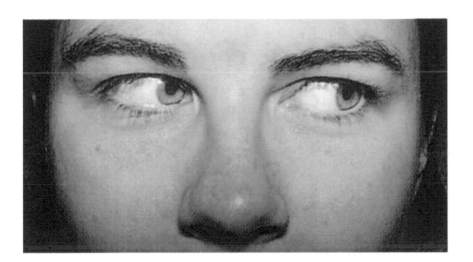

A 38-year-old woman complains of recurrent eye inflammation over the past 6 months. She says topical antibiotic drops prescribed by her internist for conjunctivitis have helped, but her eyes still feel uncomfortable and swollen.

1. What condition does the photo demonstrate that can be associated with her symptoms?

Additional information: inspection of her eyelids reveals the following:

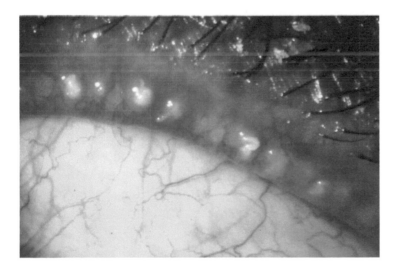

2. Describe the findings.
3. What is the diagnosis?
4. What are the types of blepharitis?
5. What are the signs of anterior blepharitis?
6. What are the treatment options for this patient?

1. Her facial appearance shows acne rosacea; ocular involvement occurs in > 50%.

2. Inflamed, obstructed Meibomian glands; pouting Meibomian gland orifices; thickened, opaque meibum; and telangiectasia of the lid margin.

3. MGD, posterior blepharitis, meibomitis.

4. Blepharitis is classified by location: anterior (infectious), posterior (MGD), and angular (lateral canthus); or etiology: chronic *Staphylococcus* or *Demodex* infection, seborrhea (alone, with staphylococcal superinfection, with meibomian seborrhea, with secondary meibomitis), primary meibomitis, atopic dermatitis, psoriasis, and fungal; angular blepharitis is associated with *Moraxella* infection.

5. Debris at the base of the eyelashes (scurf and collarettes), lid margin erythema, loss of eyelashes, conjunctival injection; sequelae include pannus, phlyctenules, corneal infiltrates and ulcers.

6. Treatment for MGD includes lid hygiene (hot compresses, lid massage, and lid scrubs or hypochlorous acid solution [Avenova, HypoChlor, Acuicyn]), oral doxycycline or minocycline, oral fish oil supplements (omega-3 fatty acids), topical azithromycin, topical steroids, topical cyclosporine, lubricating drops (for associated dry eye), heat treatment (LipiFlow, TearCare, IPL, iLux), and intraductal Meibomian gland probing. The patient may also benefit from treatment for acne rosacea.

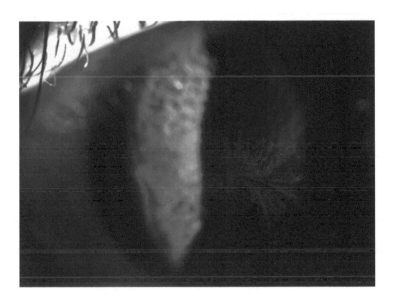

A 52-year-old woman is seen for a routine eye exam and noted to have the finding shown in the photo.

1. What is the diagnosis?
2. What is the etiology?
3. What symptoms would the patient likely have?
4. What other substances can deposit in the cornea?

1. Cornea verticillata (vortex keratopathy).

2. Fabry disease (X-linked recessive; including female carriers) and medications (systemic amiodarone, chloroquine, indomethacin, ibuprofen, naproxen, chlorpromazine, suramin, clofazimine, tamoxifen, topical netarsudil).

3. None; the deposits are asymptomatic.

4. Calcium (band keratopathy), copper (chalcosis, Wilson disease), cysteine (cystinosis), iron (from tears or hyphema), ink (corneal tattoo), lipid/cholesterol (dyslipoproteinemias), melanin, tyrosine (tyrosinemia), urate (gout), other medications (epinephrine (topical), ciprofloxacin (topical q1-2 hour), silver (argyrosis), gold (chrysiasis), mercury (topical drop preservative), thorazine/stelazine).

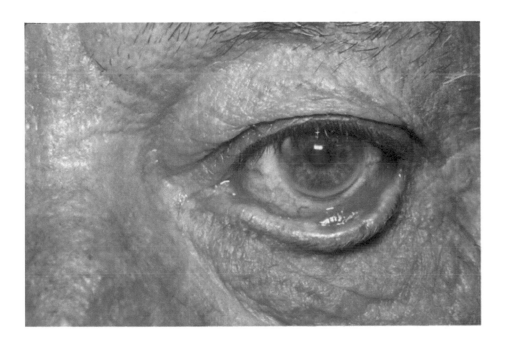

A 73-year-old man complains of redness and tearing from his left eye.

1. What is the diagnosis?

2. What are the possible etiologies?

3. How would you work up this patient?

4. What is the treatment?

1. Ectropion.

2. Cicatricial, congenital, inflammatory, involutional, mechanical, and paralytic.

3. Additional history about eye surgery, trauma, burns, infection, or facial droop (ie, Bell's palsy) should be obtained to help determine the cause of the ectropion. Examination of the lids and adnexae with respect to orbicularis function, lateral canthal tendon laxity (snap-back test, distraction test), herniated fat, and scarring will also aid in establishing the etiology. It is important to carefully inspect the inferior tarsal and bulbar conjunctiva and the cornea for signs of dryness/inflammation from exposure.

4. Ectropion-related corneal and conjunctival exposure is treated with topical lubrication (artificial tears, gel, and ointment). Treatment of the eyelid malposition depends on the etiology:

   Cicatricial: cicatrix revision/relaxation, horizontal tightening, may require vertical lengthening with full-thickness graft.

   Congenital: same as cicatricial but usually not required.

   Inflammatory: treat underlying condition.

   Involutional: horizontal shortening (lateral tarsal strip), lateral canthoplasty, repair of lower eyelid retractors.

   Mechanical: treat underlying condition.

   Paralytic: usually resolves within 6 months (Bell's palsy), otherwise lateral tarsorrhaphy, horizontal tightening, hard palate mucosal graft for lower eyelid elevation, upper eyelid gold weight implantation to improve closure.

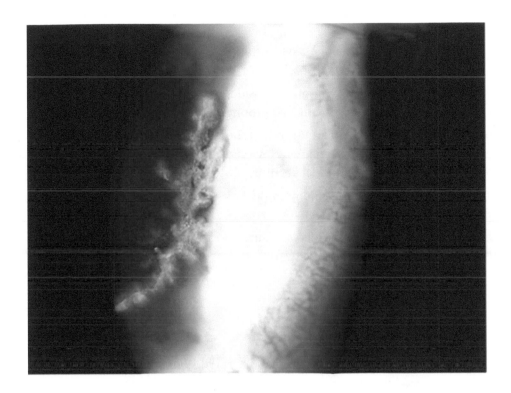

A 27-year-old man complains of acute eye pain, redness, and decreased vision for 3 days.

1. What abnormality is shown, and what is the most likely diagnosis?
2. What is the differential diagnosis of dendritic keratitis?
3. What is the treatment of HSV epithelial keratitis?
4. What is the HEDS recommendation for treatment of HSV stromal keratitis?
5. What are the complications of HSV keratitis?
6. How else can this disease manifest in the eye?

1. Corneal dendrite; HSV epithelial keratitis.

2. Herpes simplex, herpes zoster, *Acanthamoeba*, tyrosinemia, Thygeson superficial punctate keratitis, healing epithelial defect, topical prostaglandin analog toxicity.

3. Topical antiviral (Zirgan has less corneal toxicity than Viroptic), consider oral antiviral (acyclovir, famciclovir, or valacyclovir). For recurrent HSV keratitis, consider prophylaxis with long-term oral antiviral.

4. Treatment with topical steroids and Viroptic is better than Viroptic alone, and concomitant oral acyclovir has no additional benefit for the treatment of stromal keratitis. However, oral acyclovir reduces the risk of recurrent ocular disease, especially for patients with stromal keratitis.

5. Uveitis, glaucoma, episcleritis, scleritis, corneal scarring and neovascularization, corneal perforation, iris atrophy, and punctal stenosis (from topical antiviral drugs).

6. In addition to primary epithelial keratitis and various forms of recurrent keratitis, HSV may also cause vesicular blepharitis, follicular conjunctivitis, uveitis, and retinitis.

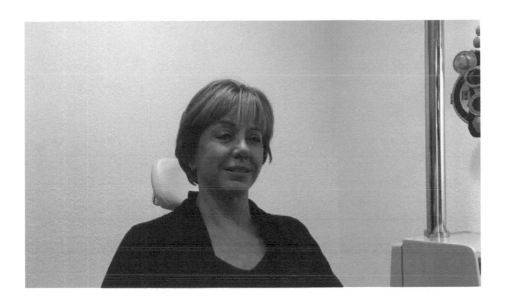

A 61-year-old woman complains that her eyes water. She has difficulty reading for more than 20 minutes at a time because of tearing and blurry vision, and at other times her eyes burn.

1. How would you evaluate this patient?
2. What specific tests are helpful?

1. Tearing, burning, and blurred vision are common symptoms of DED, so it is important to differentiate from other ocular surface disorders (blepharitis, allergic conjunctivitis) and other causes of tearing (ie, eyelid malposition, punctal stenosis, nasolacrimal duct obstruction, conjunctivochalasis). The correct diagnosis is determined with a detailed history of her symptoms (quality, timing, duration, exacerbating and ameliorating factors; consider using a questionnaire [OSDI, DEQ, NEI VFQ-25, McMonnies]), previous treatment, past ocular (particularly contact lens wear and previous eye or lid surgery) and medical (especially autoimmune disorders) histories, and medications, as well as a careful exam of the lids, lashes, conjunctiva, cornea, and tear film.

2. Surface staining with vital dyes (lissamine green or rose bengal for conjunctiva and cornea, fluorescein for cornea), height of tear meniscus, tear breakup time, tear production (Schirmer test, phenol red thread test), tear osmolarity, tear MMP-9 level; also tear lactoferrin and lysozyme levels and impression cytology. Corneal topography or keratometry may show dry spots and irregularity.

Additional information: upon further questioning she reports chronic eye irritation for years, worse at the end of the day and after long periods of working on the computer. She can no longer wear contact lenses comfortably and only gets temporary relief from lubricating drops, which she uses several times a day. She denies any ocular surgery or trauma and does not have any allergies. Her medical history is notable for hypertension for which she takes hydrochlorothiazide. Slit lamp exam shows:

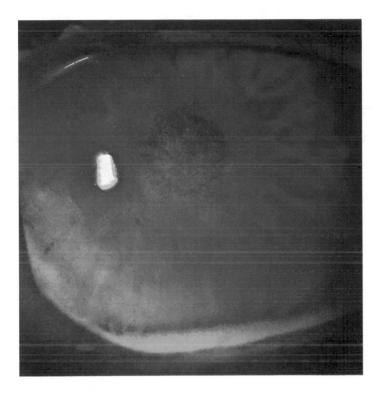

3. How is dry eye classified?
4. What are the treatment options?

3. DED can be classified by mechanism (decreased tear production or increased tear evaporation), category (lid margin disease [ie, blepharitis, meibomitis], no lid margin disease, altered tear distribution/clearance), or severity. The most common classification is aqueous deficient (abnormal lacrimal gland function resulting in decreased tear production) or evaporative (normal lacrimal gland function but increased tear evaporation because of lipid or mucin deficiency). Most cases of dry eye are multifactorial, and approximately 86% of patients with dry eye have signs of MGD.

Aqueous deficient: Sjogren syndrome and non-Sjogren syndrome (age-related, intrinsic lacrimal gland deficiency, lacrimal gland inflammation and infiltration, lacrimal gland obstruction, hyposecretory states, other disorders).

Evaporative: lid-related (MGD, disorders of lid aperture, congruity, dynamics) and ocular surface-related (allergic eye disease, vitamin A deficiency, iatrogenic).

The DEWS report classified DED by severity level (based on symptoms and signs) and recommended treatments accordingly:

Level 1: mild symptoms, mild conjunctival signs, no staining.

Level 2: moderate symptoms, tear film and visual signs, conjunctival staining, mild corneal staining.

Level 3: severe symptoms, marked corneal staining, filamentary keratitis.

Level 4: extremely severe symptoms, severe corneal staining, corneal erosions, conjunctival scarring.

4. Treatment depends on the severity of disease. Any underlying condition must also be treated. The DEWS II recommendations include:

Step 1: education, reduce/eliminate associated factors, lubrication (artificial tears, gels, ointments, lacrisert), nutritional supplements (omega-3 fatty acids), lid hygiene and warm compresses.

Step 2: non-preserved lubricants, punctal plug, moisture chamber goggles, humidifier, topical steroids (short duration), cyclosporine (Restasis, Cequa), lifitegrast (Xiidra), acetylcysteine (Mucomyst), secretogogues, topical antibiotic or antibiotic/steroid combination for anterior blepharitis, oral macrolide or tetracyclines, meibomian gland heating and expression treatments (ie, LipiFlow, TearCare, IPL, iLux) for MGD, tea tree oil for *Demodex*, neurostimulation device (iTear100).

Step 3: oral secretogogues, autologous serum drops, therapeutic contact lens (soft bandage, rigid scleral Boston ocular surface prosthesis (PROSE lens).

Step 4: topical steroid (long duration), amniotic membrane grafts, permanent punctal occlusion, other surgery (tarsorraphy, mucous membrane, salivary gland transplantation).

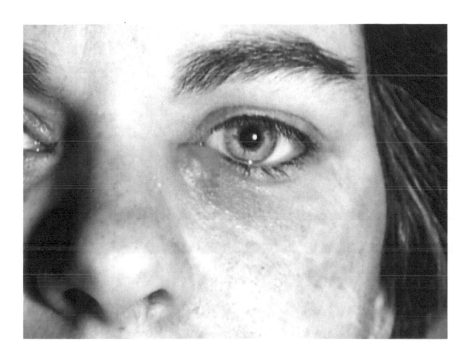

A 58-year-old woman reports a swollen left lower eyelid for the past 5 days. She has used warm compresses, but the swelling has gotten worse and the area is painful. She denies any change in vision. Her past ocular history is negative except for an occasional stye when she was a teenager.

1. Describe the abnormality?
2. What is the differential diagnosis?

Additional information: she has no history of sinus or upper respiratory infection, and there is no history of trauma. Palpation under the medial canthal tendon produces discharge from the punctum. The eye exam is otherwise normal.

3. What is the most likely diagnosis?
4. What is the etiology?
5. How would you treat this patient?

1. Erythema and swelling of the lower eyelid at the medial canthus.

2. Hordeolum, cellulitis, abscess, ethmoid sinusitis, lacrimal sac tumor.

3. Acute dacryocystitis.

4. Bacterial infection (*Streptococcus pneumoniae, Staphylococcus, Pseudomonas; Haemophilus influenzae* [in children]). Predisposing conditions (causing lacrimal sac tear stasis) include strictures, long/narrow nasolacrimal duct, lacrimal sac diverticulum, trauma, dacryoliths, nasolacrimal duct obstruction, inflammatory sinus and nasal disorders.

5. Culture and Gram stain of lacrimal sac contents (percutaneous aspirate), systemic antibiotics (Augmentin or Bactrim for 10 days), and continue warm compresses several times a day. A pointing abscess can be incised and drained. Consider dacryocystorhinostomy after the infection resolves.

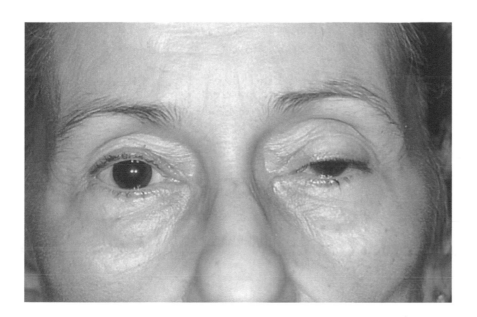

A 71-year-old woman says her eyes feel tired and notices a droopy eyelid.

1. What is the differential diagnosis?
2. How is ptosis classified?
3. What measurements are helpful?

Additional information: she has good levator function and is diagnosed with aponeurotic ptosis.

4. What is the treatment?

1. Blepharoptosis, dermatochalasis (excess skin of upper eyelids; pseudoptosis), lid swelling, lid tumor, enophthalmos, hypotropioa, contralateral eyelid retraction or proptosis, and small eye.

2. Ptosis is classified by etiology:

   Aponeurotic (involutional): most common form of ptosis caused by disinsertion, central dehiscence, or attenuation of the levator aponeurosis. Associated with age, eye surgery, ocular trauma, pregnancy, chronic eyelid swelling, and blepharochalasis; good levator function.

   Mechanical: caused by mass effect (tumors) or scarring (cicatricial ptosis); good levator function.

   Myogenic: weakness of levator palpebrae superioris caused by muscular disorders (chronic progressive external ophthalmoplegia, myotonic dystrophy, and oculopharyngeal dystrophy); extremely poor levator function.

   Neurogenic: caused by defects in innervation to cranial nerve III (oculomotor palsy) or sympathetic input to Müller muscle (Horner syndrome) or generalized dysfunction of neuromuscular junction (myasthenia gravis); variable levator function depending on etiology.

   Congenital: usually myogenic with fibrosis and fat infiltration of levator muscle, but can also be caused by aponeurosis dehiscence (possibly birth trauma), congenital Horner syndrome (ptosis, miosis, anhidrosis, iris hypopigmentation) with poor Müller muscle function from decreased sympathetic tone, or congenital neurogenic with Marcus Gunn jaw-winking syndrome from aberrant connections between cranial nerve V (innervating the pterygoid muscles) and the levator muscle.

3. Eyelid measurements include margin reflex distance (MRD1, distance between upper eyelid margin and corneal light reflex, normal is 4.5 mm; MRD2, distance between lower eyelid margin and corneal light reflex, normal is 5 mm), palpebral fissure height (PF, distance between upper and lower eyelid margins; MRD1 + MRD2), upper lid crease height (distance from upper eyelid margin to lid crease in downgaze; normal is 6-8 mm in men and 8-10 mm in women; high in aponeurotic ptosis), and levator function (LF, distance the upper lid margin travels between downgaze and upgaze; normal is 13-17 mm).

4. Surgical repair with levator aponeurosis advancement, levator resection, muellerectomy, or Fasanella–Servat tarsoconjunctival resection. Consider medical treatment for mild cases or to temporize prior to surgery with topical α-agonist (Upneeq or Alphagan).

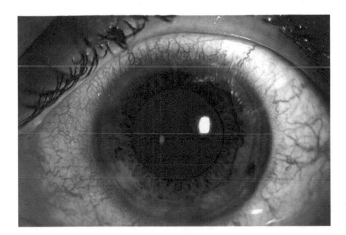

A 31-year-old woman complains of red, irritated eyes for 5 days.

1. What is the differential diagnosis?
2. What questions would you ask her?

Additional information: she reports having a recent cold and denies any trauma, allergies, inciting event, contact lens wear, or previous episodes. The symptoms started OD with redness, burning, morning crusting, and sticky tears. There was lid swelling and OS involvement the following day. She has used Visine and cold compresses for the last 3 days with minimal effect. On exam, her vision is 20/30 OD and 20/25 OS, there is 2+ conjunctival injection, and inferior tarsal follicles OU. Slit lamp photo of the cornea shows:

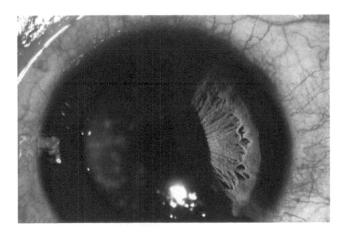

3. What is the corneal finding?
4. What is the diagnosis?
5. What is the causative organism?
6. What other infections does this organism cause?
7. How would you treat this patient?

1. Conjunctivitis (infectious, allergic, other), dry eye disease, blepharitis, Meibomian gland dysfunction, conjunctival or corneal foreign body or abrasion, episcleritis, iritis.

2. What is the nature of the irritation (burning, stinging, itching, foreign body sensation)? Was there any inciting factor or trauma? Does she suffer from allergies? Has she had a recent URI, been in contact with anyone with an eye infection, wear contact lenses? Is there any discharge? If so, what type? Does she have crusting of the eyelashes in the morning? Any decrease in vision? Has she used any treatment? Has this happened before? Is she taking any new medications?

3. SEIs.

4. EKC.

5. Adenovirus. There are 7 subgroups (A–G) and > 52 serotypes, 1/3 are associated with eye infection (majority are group D). Types 8, 19 (reclassified as 64), and 37 are most severe, and types 53, 54, and 56 are less severe. Many types also cause nonspecific follicular conjunctivitis.

6. Respiratory and gastrointestinal.

7. Treatment is supportive with lubrication, hot compresses (to remove crusting) and cold compresses (to relieve swelling and discomfort), topical vasoconstrictor, antihistamine, mast cell stabilizer, NSAID for redness and irritation. Consider a course of topical ganciclovir gel (Zirgan), hypochlorous acid, or in office one-time application of povidone-iodine 5% ophthalmic solution. Topical steroids or cyclosporine may be used to reduce severe inflammation and for SEIs.

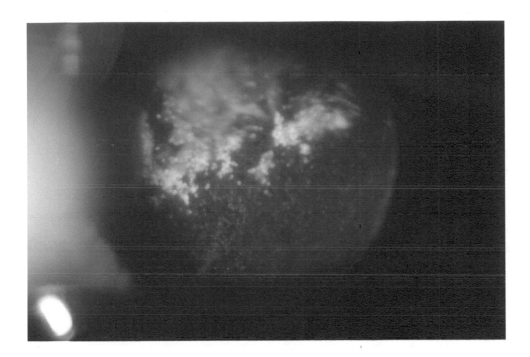

A 72-year-old woman 3 months status post uncomplicated cataract surgery in the left eye complains of blurry vision for 2 weeks. The cornea is clear, there is a mild anterior chamber reaction, and the IOL is centered in the bag.

1. What is the differential diagnosis?
2. What are the characteristic signs of chronic endophthalmitis?
3. What is the most likely causative organism?
4. How would you confirm the diagnosis?

Additional information: the culture is positive for Propionibacterium acnes.

5. What is the treatment?

1. Intraocular inflammation due to rebound iritis, retained lens material, or delayed-onset/chronic endophthalmitis.

2. Posterior capsular plaque, iritis, keratic precipitates, may have keratitis, hypopyon, mild vitritis, and cystoid macular edema.

3. *Propionibacterium acnes*, coagulase-negative *Staphylococcus*, or fungi (*Candida* or *Aspergillus*). Other rarer organisms include *Actinomycetes* and *Nocardia*.

4. Anterior chamber tap for culture and smear is often negative, so diagnosis usually requires culturing the plaque on the posterior capsule.

5. *Propionibacterium acnes* endophthalmitis treated with only intraocular vancomycin and topical steroids is often unsuccessful. It usually also requires a vitrectomy, injection of vancomycin into the capsular bag, partial or total capsulectomy, and IOL removal or exchange.

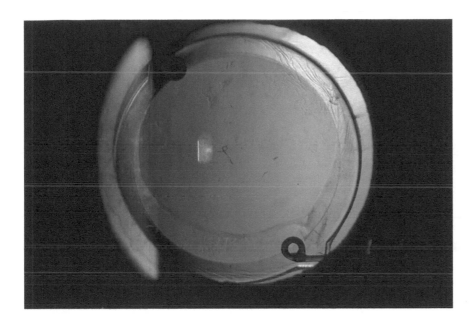

An 84-year-old man with aphakia OD and pseudophakia OS wears a rigid gas permeable contact lens OD, which gives him 20/25 vision. However, he finds it increasingly difficult to insert and remove the contact lens, so he is interested in surgery.

1. What are the secondary IOL options?
2. How would you determine where to place the lens?
3. What other findings are important to note for planning the surgical procedure?

Additional information: the patient has a large corneoscleral wound superiorly with thinning. The cornea is clear without guttata, there is a sector iridectomy superiorly, and some peripheral capsule is visible. The angle is open with scattered PAS, and there is a small knuckle of vitreous prolapsing into the anterior chamber.

4. What surgical technique would you recommend?
5. What are the disadvantages of a scleral-sutured IOL?

1. Secondary IOL in the bag, sulcus (with or without suture fixation to the iris or sclera), iris-fixated, or anterior chamber.

2. Placement depends on anatomic factors, health of the eye, patient's general health, and surgeon preference/comfort. It is important to assess the status of the cornea, angle, any remaining lens capsule, macula, peripheral retina, and optic nerve. Can the patient tolerate a lengthy procedure? Is the patient on anticoagulation?

3. Location of previous cataract wound, presence of iridectomy, posterior synechiae to capsule, amount and stability of any capsule, and vitreous in the anterior chamber.

4. A sulcus lens possibly with suture support or an iris-fixated IOL is the only choice since there is no intact capsule in the bag placement and there are PAS, which is a contraindication for an anterior chamber IOL. Because of the thinning at the superior limbus from the previous surgical wound, a temporal incision is preferred for this case. An anterior vitrectomy must be performed first to clear all vitreous anterior to the capsular plane. For unsutured sulcus placement, it is necessary to assess the remaining capsule for adequacy of supporting a posterior chamber IOL. If support appears to be sufficient, then a foldable three-piece or rigid one-piece IOL can be placed in the sulcus. The IOL stability must be tested by decentering the IOL in various meridians and observing for spontaneous recentration. If the IOL is not stable, then suture fixation to the iris may be performed. If it initially appears that capsular support is inadequate, then the IOL can be sutured to the iris or to the sclera or fixated to sclera with tunnel placement and fibrin glue or cautery (terminal bulb/flange formation). Alternatively, an iris-fixated (iris-claw) lens can be used. After placement of the IOL, the sector iridectomy can be repaired with McCannel sutures. These sutures can be tied externally or internally using the Siepser technique.

5. It is technically more difficult, takes more time, and requires a thorough anterior vitrectomy. The main risks are long-term stability and damage to uveal tissue. Other complications include IOL tilt, IOL decentration, pigment dispersion, uveitis, intraocular hemorrhage (hyphema, vitreous hemorrhage, choroidal hemorrhage), suture exposure or erosion, endophthalmitis, CME, and retinal detachment. Numerous techniques have been developed to minimize these risks.

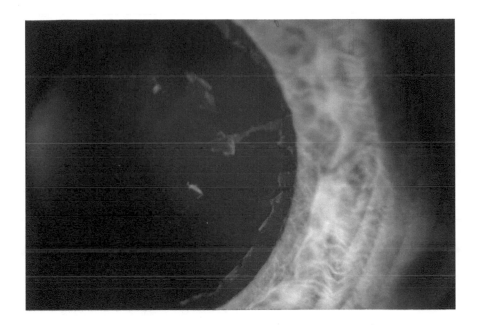

A 67-year-old man has a visually significant cataract and desires surgery. On exam, he dilates poorly and his lens appearance is seen in the photo.

1. What condition does he have and what other ocular problems are associated with it?
2. What other history would be helpful?

Additional information: the patient has a history of increased IOP, but has not been treated. His only medical condition is arthritis for which he takes ibuprofen as needed.

3. What would you pay particular attention to on exam?
4. What specific risks does this patient have with respect to cataract surgery?

1. PXS, which is associated with angle closure, ectopia lentis, ocular hypertension, and PXG.

2. What is his past ocular and medical history? Does he have any other ocular problems or has he been treated for any eye conditions? What medications does he take? Specifically, does he take medicine for his prostate or blood pressure?

3. Gonioscopy, diameter of dilated pupil, iridodonesis, phacodonesis, corneal pachymetry, IOP, and optic nerve appearance.

4. He should be warned that PXS increase the chance of complications because of weak zonules. These include posterior capsular rupture, zonular dehiscence, vitreous loss, retained lens fragments, alternate lens placement, late lens dislocation, iris damage, and misshapen pupil. He should also be informed of an increased risk for PXG in the future, even if the lens is removed.

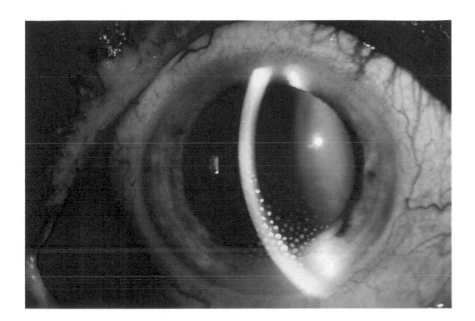

A 52-year-old asymptomatic woman comes in for a complete eye exam. An anterior segment exam shows the finding in the photo. A posterior segment exam shows mild attenuation of the retinal vasculature and diffuse pigmentary changes in both eyes.

1.   What questions would you ask her?

Additional information: she reports a few episodes of "conjunctivitis" for which she was given antibiotic and steroid drops. Cultures or additional workup were not performed. Her past medical history is positive for Chlamydia at age 28 and hypercholesterolemia.

2.   What would you do next?

Additional information: the tests are negative except for a positive VDRL and FTA-ABS.

3.   What treatment would you prescribe and why?
4.   What is the organism?
5.   What other ocular findings occur in this disease?
6.   What are the systemic signs of congenital syphilis?

1. Does she have any past ocular history (disease, infection, trauma)? Has she ever had an episode of a red eye with blurry vision or photophobia? Is there any past medical history, specifically arthritis, autoimmune disorders, or infectious disease? Has she ever had a sexually transmitted disease?

2. The patient has had bilateral uveitis and requires a workup including CBC, RF, ANA, ACE, VDRL or RPR, FTA-ABS or MHA-TP, PPD and controls, and CXR.

3. Lumbar puncture to rule out neurosyphilis, and treat the patient and all sexual partners with systemic penicillin (or tetracycline if allergic to penicillin). Follow serum VDRL or RPR to monitor treatment efficacy.

4. *Treponema pallidum*, a spirochete.

5. Interstitial keratitis, uveitis, ectopia lentis, Argyll–Robertson pupil, chorioretinitis, and optic atrophy.

6. Hutchinson teeth (peg-shaped), mulberry molars, saber shins, saddle nose, frontal bossing, deafness, tabes dorsalis, skin fissures (rhagades; especially corners of mouth and nose), internal organ inflammation, neurosyphilis.

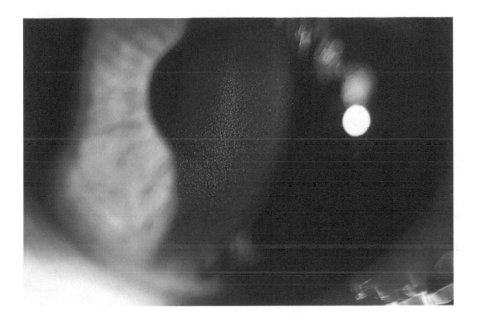

A 37-year-old man wants a new glasses prescription.

1. What finding is depicted in the photo?

2. What is the diagnosis?

3. What other findings would you expect to see?

4. What are the ocular associations?

5. If this patient develops high IOP requiring treatment, what would you recommend?

6. What is the pathophysiology?

7. What is the mechanism of glaucoma?

8. What is the natural course of the condition?

1. Krukenberg spindle.

2. PDS or PG.

3. Heavily pigmented trabecular meshwork, radial midperipheral iris transillumination defects, pigment in iris furrows and on anterior lens capsule, iridodonesis, may have increased IOP (IOP spikes with blurry vision and halos may occur from exercise or pupil dilation), optic nerve cupping, and visual field defects.

4. Myopia, lattice degeneration (20%), PG develops in up to 50% of patients with PDS.

5. PDS/PG tends to respond well to laser trabeculoplasty, so this may be a better initial choice than using a topical medication (with associated side effects and cost) indefinitely. Miotics (ie, pilocarpine) minimize the iris–zonule touch.

6. The iris has a concave configuration with contact against the zonules. Iris movement causes pigment liberation from the posterior surface as it rubs against the underlying zonules during normal pupillary movement. Factors associated with concave iris contour include posterior iris insertion, accommodation, and blinking, which also increases the pressure gradient from the anterior to posterior chamber causing more posterior iris bowing and iridolenticular contact (reverse pupillary block).

7. PG is a secondary open-angle glaucoma in which iris pigment obstructs the trabecular meshwork causing elevated IOP and optic nerve damage.

8. PDS usually burns itself out because once all the pigment has been liberated, there is no more to clog the trabecular meshwork and raise the IOP.

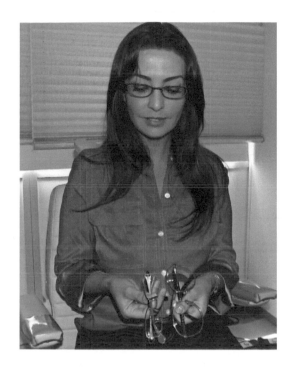

A 46-year-old woman complains that her distance vision has gotten worse over the past year and she has needed frequent changes in the left lens of her glasses.

1.   What is the differential diagnosis?

Additional information: she has no past ocular or medical history and she does not take any medication.

2.   If her routine ophthalmic exam appears normal, what other ocular testing would you perform?

Additional information: further exam shows increased cylinder on refraction, normal corneal topography and gonioscopy, and a segmental cataract in the left eye.

3.   What is the most likely diagnosis, differential diagnosis, and what test would you use to confirm it?
4.   This patient has a ciliary body melanoma. What other findings may occur?
5.   What is the distribution of uveal melanoma?
6.   What is the treatment?
7.   What is the prognosis?

1. The change in refractive error is due to induced myopia, hyperopia, or astigmatism, which can result from systemic or ocular conditions. The differential diagnosis is:

    Acquired myopia:

    > **Increased lens power:** nuclear sclerotic cataract, change in lens position or shape (medication [miotics]), anterior lens dislocation, excessive accommodation), osmotic effect (diabetes, galactosemia, uremia, sulfonamides), anterior lenticonus.

    > **Increased corneal power:** keratoconus, contact lens-induced corneal warpage, congenital glaucoma.

    > **Increased axial length:** posterior staphyloma, after scleral buckle surgery, congenital glaucoma, retinopathy of prematurity.

    Acquired hyperopia:

    > **Decreased refractive power:** lens change (posterior lens dislocation, aphakia, diabetes), drugs (chloroquine, phenothiazines, antihistamines, benzodiazepines), poor accommodation (tonic pupil, drugs, trauma), flattening of cornea (contact lens, radial keratotomy surgery), intraocular silicone oil.

    > **Decreased effective axial length:** retrobulbar tumor, choroidal tumor, central serous chorioretinopathy, posterior scleritis, serous retinal detachment.

    Acquired astigmatism:

    > Lid lesion (tumor, chalazion, ptosis), pterygium, limbal dermoid, corneal degenerations and ectasias, surgery (corneal, cataract), lenticular, ciliary body tumor.

2. Corneal topography, gonioscopy, transillumination, UBM, OCT, B-scan ultrasound.

3. Ciliary body tumor, for which the differential diagnosis is iridociliary epithelial cyst, foreign body granuloma, nevus, melanocytoma, malignant melanoma, leiomyoma, Fuchs adenoma, sarcoid nodule, and metastasis. Visualization can be achieved with UBM, anterior segment OCT, or Scheimpflug imaging.

4. In addition to lenticular astigmatism and cataract, signs of ciliary body melanoma include shallow anterior chamber, sentinel vessel, and extrascleral extension.

5. Malignant melanoma of the uveal tract involves the choroid (90%), ciliary body (6%), and iris (4%).

6. Depending on the extent of the tumor, treatment is with surgical excision, chemotherapy, radiation, or enucleation.

7. The prognosis is poorer than for iris melanoma because ciliary body melanoma is usually diagnosed at a later stage. The risk of metastasis is 25% at 5 years, 34% at 10 years, and 55% at 20 years.

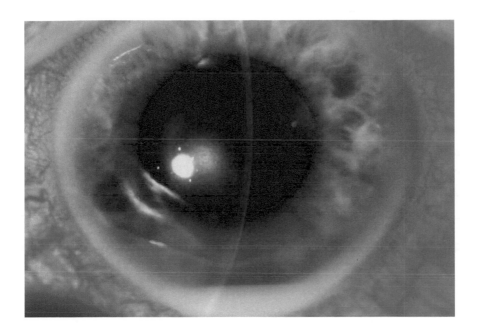

A 50-year-old man presents with a recurrence of acute anterior uveitis and reports multiple episodes over the past 15 years. He denies any eye injury or surgery. Exam of the involved eye shows 20/40 vision, ciliary flush, 2+ anterior chamber cells and flare, hypopyon, fine keratic precipitates, and no vitreous cells.

1. What additional history would be helpful?
2. What other findings would you look for on exam?
3. What is the differential diagnosis?

Additional information: the patient has no significant past medical history. He denies ocular herpes. He has eczema and occasional back pain, and he takes NSAIDs as needed. He travels internationally several times a year. IOP and gonioscopy are normal.

4. What targeted workup would you order?
5. What disorders are associated with HLA-B27 iritis?
6. What is the treatment for this patient's acute iritis?
7. What are the possible complications of iritis?

1. Past medical history, medication history, and review of systems with attention to joint pain, skin changes/ rashes, infections, oral lesions, urethritis, genital ulcers, diarrhea, foreign travel, and conjunctivitis.

2. Increased IOP, corneal edema, corneal scarring, synechiae, iris color, iris atrophy, cataract, and CME.

3. The differential diagnosis of nongranulomatous iritis is idiopathic, HLA-B27 associated, Fuchs heterochromic iridocyclitis, HSV, glaucomatocyclitic crisis (Posner–Schlossman syndrome), Lyme disease, Behçet disease, drugs, and interstitial nephritis.

4. This patient most likely has iritis associated with HLA-B27, so a targeted approach would be to order HLA-B27, sacroiliac X-ray, CBC with differential, urinalysis, VDRL or RPR, and FTA-ABS or MHA-TP.

5. Ankylosing spondylitis, reactive arthritis syndrome, psoriatic arthritis, inflammatory bowel disease, and Whipple disease.

6. Frequent topical steroids and cycloplegia.

7. Cataract, glaucoma, synechiae, band keratopathy, iris atrophy, CME.

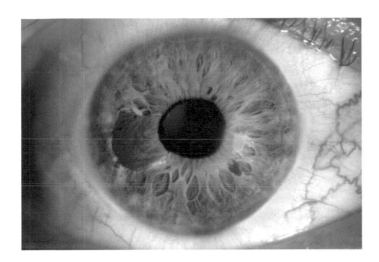

A 61-year-old woman says that her blue eye is turning brown.

1. What is the differential diagnosis?

2. On clinical exam, how is a nevus differentiated from a melanoma?

3. What are the risk factors for malignant transformation of an iris nevus?

4. If you suspect a melanoma, what tests may be helpful?

Additional information: the pathology shows:

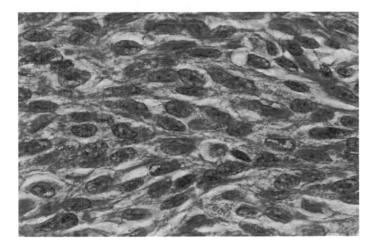

5. What is the diagnosis?

6. What are the various presentations of this disease?

7. How is iris melanoma classified?

8. What is the treatment?

9. What is the prognosis?

1. A pigmented iris lesion could be a nevus, melanocytoma, melanoma, iris pigment epithelial tumor, or rarely metastasis (usually amelanotic).

2. An iris nevus can be distinguished from a melanoma by: size (<3 mm in diameter), thickness (<1 mm thick), and the absence of vascularity, ectropion uveae, secondary cataract, secondary glaucoma, and growth.

3. Mnemonic **ABCDEF**: **A**ge (<40 years), **B**lood (hyphema), **C**lock hour inferiorly (4:00–9:00), **D**iffuse appearance, **E**ctropion uveae, **F**eathery margins. Risk of suspicious nevus progressing to melanoma is 4% in 10 years and 11% in 20 years.

4. Iris FA (a nevus has a filigree filling pattern that becomes hyperfluorescent early and leaks late or is angiographically silent, whereas a malignant melanoma has irregular vessels that fill late), and B-scan ultrasound or UBM to rule out ciliary body involvement. Transillumination may also be helpful.

5. Malignant melanoma (spindle cell).

6. An iris malignant melanoma may be diffuse (associated with heterochromia and secondary glaucoma), tapioca (dark tapioca appearance), ring shaped, or localized. It may have feeder vessels, involve angle structures, cause sectoral cataract, hyphema, increased IOP, or glaucoma.

7. *American Joint Cancer Committee classification:*

   T1: limited to iris (1a = ≤3 clock hours, 1b = >3 clock hours, 1c = with secondary glaucoma)

   T2: confluent with or extending into ciliary body, choroid, or both (2a = ciliary body without secondary glaucoma, 2b = ciliary body and choroid without secondary glaucoma, 2c = ciliary body, choroid, or both with secondary glaucoma)

   T3: T2 with scleral extension

   T4: with extrasceral extension (4a = ≤5 mm in diameter, 4b = >5 mm in diameter)

8. Treatment includes chemotherapy, radiation, complete surgical excision, and enucleation depending on the extent. The patient may need treatment of increased IOP.

9. The prognosis is good especially for small tumors. The risk of mortality is 3%; 5% metastasis at 5 years, 7% at 10 years, and 11% at 20 years. The risk of metastasis is increased if there is elevated IOP or extraocular extension.

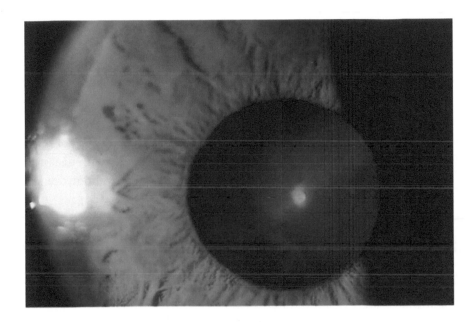

A 66-year-old hyperopic man with BCVA of 20/60 OD and 20/30 OS desires cataract surgery in both eyes.

1. What additional history and testing would you obtain to determine if he is a suitable candidate for surgery in the left eye?

2. What are the etiologies and symptoms associated with this type of cataract?

3. What are the medical indications for cataract surgery?

4. The patient is extremely anxious and wants general anesthesia for the phacoemulsification procedure. You decide to use monitored anesthesia care and a retrobulbar block. What are the possible complications of a retrobulbar injection?

5. During surgery, the patient starts to cough. What complications can result from this?

6. During IOL implantation, a darkening of the red reflex is seen, the iris prolapses, and the IOL cannot be placed in the bag due to vitreous pressure. What is happening?

7. How would you treat this complication?

1. How does the reduced vision interfere with his daily activities and hobbies? Does he have sensitivity to light? Is he experiencing difficulty in dimmer lighting conditions or with glare/halos from lights? Does he notice difficulty in reading? Helpful tests to perform include glare testing, near vision, pinhole vision, slit-lamp exam with attention to the type, degree, and density of the lens opacity, and the quality of the view on fundus exam.

2. Nuclear sclerotic and cortical cataracts are most commonly associated with age, ultraviolet (UV-B) exposure, and smoking. Both types of cataracts result in decreased and blurry vision and reduced contrast and color sensitivity. Nuclear sclerosis typically produces a myopic shift and more difficulty with distance than with near vision, whereas cortical spokes and vacuoles are more likely to cause glare and polyopia.

3. Cataracts that are causing a secondary eye disorder (ie, phacolytic, phacomorphic, or lens-particle glaucoma) or are obstructing the view of the posterior pole to the extent that they are interfering with the adequate diagnosis and treatment of retinal or optic nerve disease (ie, diabetes, macular degeneration, glaucoma).

4. Central anesthesia (from subarachnoid or intradural injection), retrobulbar hemorrhage, globe penetration or perforation, optic nerve damage (direct or indirect), ophthalmic artery occlusion, retinal vascular occlusion (vein or artery), strabismus (inferior rectus fibrosis or myotoxicity), ptosis.

5. Shallow chamber, iris prolapse, choroidal effusion/hemorrhage.

6. Choroidal effusion or suprachoroidal hemorrhage.

7. Immediately close the incision, administer mannitol, consider sclerotomies to drain blood/fluid, monitor the IOP, and implant the IOL at a later time (hours to days).

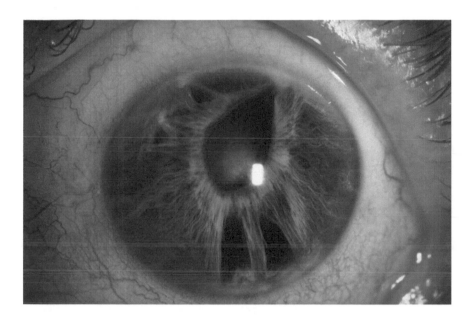

A 33-year-old woman complains of double vision and a funny looking pupil in her left eye.

1. What is the differential diagnosis of monocular diplopia?
2. What condition do you suspect she has?
3. What are the characteristic findings of each disorder in this syndrome?
4. What is the pathophysiology?

1. Uncorrected refractive error, cataract, corneal pathology (irregular astigmatism from anterior basement membrane dystrophy, scar, or ectasia), iris hole(s), rarely macular pathology.

2. ICE syndromes, specifically essential iris atrophy.

3. The 3 syndromes that comprise ICE have the common features of iris distortion, corneal edema, and secondary angle-closure glaucoma due to angle endothelialization and PAS formation. The specific findings of each syndrome are:

   Iris nevus (Cogan–Reese) syndrome: flattening and effacement of the iris stroma, pigmented iris nodules (pseudonevi) composed of normal iris cells that are bunched up from the overlying membrane, corectopia, and ectropion uveae.

   Chandler syndrome: corneal edema often with normal IOP, and mild or no iris changes (minimal corectopia, iris atrophy, PAS).

   Essential iris atrophy (progressive iris atrophy): proliferating endothelium produces broad PAS, corectopia, ectropion uveae, and iris holes (stretch holes [area away from maximal pull of endothelial membrane is stretched so thin that holes develop] and melting holes [holes in areas without iris thinning due to iris ischemia]).

4. Abnormal corneal endothelium grows across the angle and iris, obstructs the trabecular meshwork, distorts the iris, and contracts around the iris stroma to form nodules.

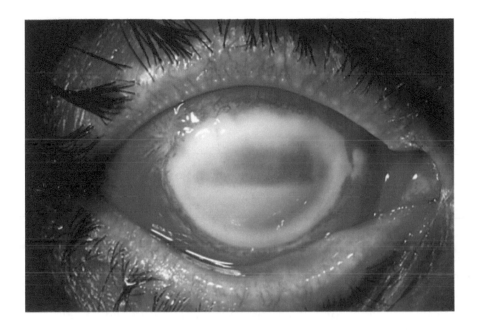

A 68-year-old woman sees you 5 days after uncomplicated cataract surgery because her eye has become progressively red and painful with blurry vision.

1. What is the diagnosis?
2. What are the most common organisms?
3. What are the risk factors?
4. What steps have been shown to reduce the risk of endophthalmitis?
5. What are the characteristic findings?
6. What are the EVS treatment recommendations?

1. Acute postoperative endophthalmitis.

2. Ninety-four percent of acute postoperative endophthalmitis is caused by Gram-positive bacteria: coagulase-negative staphylococci (70%), *Staphylococcus aureus* (10%), *Streptococcus* species (11%). Only 6% is due to Gram-negative bacteria.

3. Complicated surgery (prolonged surgical time, disrupted posterior capsule, vitreous loss, wound leak, iris prolapse), blepharitis, diabetes, immunosuppression.

4. *Preoperative*: povidone-iodine on the ocular surface, barrier draping the eyelashes.

   Intraoperative: preservative-free antibiotics in irrigating solution (ie, vancomycin) or injected intracamerally at the conclusion of surgery (ie, cefuroxime, vancomycin, or Vigamox).

5. Decreased visual acuity, lid edema, proptosis, conjunctival injection, chemosis, wound abscess, corneal edema, keratic precipitates, anterior chamber cells and flare, hypopyon, vitritis, poor red reflex, and may have positive Seidel test at wound.

6. *Better than LP vision*: anterior chamber and vitreous tap to collect specimens for culture, and intravitreal antibiotics (vancomycin and ceftazidime or amikacin). Also treat with subconjunctival (vancomycin and ceftazidime or gentamicin) and topical (fortified vancomycin and ceftazidime) antibiotics and steroids, and a topical cycloplegic. Intravitreal steroids were not evaluated, and systemic antibiotics were not found to be beneficial.

   LP vision or worse: same as above but also perform pars plana vitrectomy.

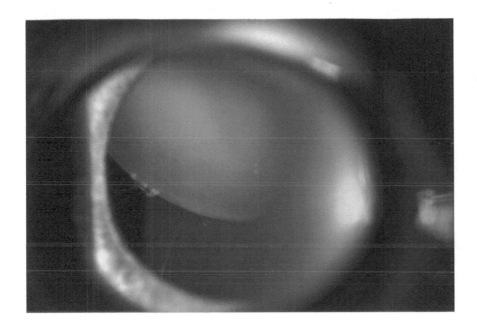

A 42-year-old man reports gradual deterioration of vision in his left eye. The slit-lamp exam is notable for the finding shown here.

1. What are the possible etiologies?
2. What are the findings of Marfan syndrome, Weill–Marchesani syndrome, homocystinuria, hyperlysinemia, and sulfite oxidase deficiency?
3. What symptoms may this patient have?
4. What are the treatment options?
5. What are the surgical techniques for lens extraction?

1. Ectopia lentis is caused by trauma (most common acquired cause), Marfan syndrome, Weill–Marchesani syndrome, Stickler syndrome, Ehlers–Danlos syndrome, homocystinuria, hyperlysinemia, sulfite oxidase deficiency, aniridia, congenital glaucoma, megalocornea, hereditary ectopia lentis, and ectopia lentis et pupillae, tertiary syphilis, congenital Zika syndrome, medulloepithelioma, pseudoexfoliation syndrome (rare).

2. *Marfan syndrome*: ectopia lentis (65%; usually superotemporal), glaucoma, keratoconus, cornea plana, axial myopia, retinal degeneration (salt and pepper fundus), retinal detachment, tall stature, disproportionate growth of extremities, arachnodactyly, joint laxity, pectus deformities, scoliosis, and increasing dilation of the ascending aorta with aortic insufficiency.

    Weill–Marchesani syndrome: ectopia lentis (usually inferiorly or anteriorly), microspherophakia, high lenticular myopia, cataract, microcornea, glaucoma (pupillary block), short stature, stubby fingers with broad hands, hearing defects, inflexible joints, mental retardation.

    Homocystinuria: bilateral ectopia lentis (90% usually inferonasal; 30% in infancy, 80% by age 15 years), enlarged globe, myopia, peripheral retinal pigment epithelium degeneration, retinal detachment, early loss of accommodation, blonde hair, tall (marfinoid habitus with arachnodactyly), osteoporosis, fractures, seizures, mental retardation (50%), cardiomegaly, platelet abnormality with hypercoagulability (thromboembolism), 75% mortality by age 30 years.

    Hyperlysinemia: ectopia lentis, microspherophakia, and growth, motor and mental retardation.

    Sulfite oxidase deficiency: ectopia lentis (50%), enophthalmos, Brushfield spots, seizures, mental retardation, frontal bossing.

3. Blurry vision due to induced refractive error, diplopia if the lens equator is in the visual axis, and may have symptoms of angle-closure glaucoma.

4. Glasses or contact lens for refractive error, miotics for diplopia, and consider lens extraction. Patients may require treatment of angle-closure glaucoma and any underlying disorder.

5. Phacoemulsification (with capsular support system and sutured capsular rings or ring segments for IOL placement in the bag, otherwise sulcus IOL with or without suture fixation, iris-fixated IOL, or anterior chamber IOL, and may require anterior vitrectomy) by anterior segment surgeon or lensectomy/vitrectomy by retinal surgeon depending on the degree of lens displacement and instability.

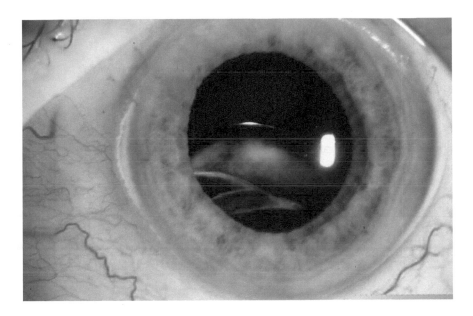

A 79-year-old woman with pseudoexfoliation syndrome status post uncomplicated cataract surgery 6 years ago notices increasing blurry vision after bumping her forehead on a towel rack in the bathroom 2 weeks ago.

1. What is the term for the finding demonstrated in the photo?
2. What are the etiologies?
3. How would you treat a subluxed IOL?

1. Sunset syndrome.

2. *In the bag IOL:* zonulolysis from trauma or any other condition that can cause ectopia lentis (see Case 119).

   Sulcus IOL: insufficient capsular support, inappropriate IOL (length too short for sulcus), capsular contraction with asymmetric haptic placement (one in and one out of bag).

3. IOL repositioning or exchange. For repositioning, the haptics (or capsular tension ring if present) can be sewn to the iris or sclera using a variety of techniques. For exchange, depending on the adequacy of capsular support and the status of the anterior chamber, the lens options are a sulcus IOL (with or without suture fixation), an iris-fixated IOL, and an anterior chamber IOL.

A 74-year-old man says he has pain in his left eye and forehead and blurry vision for 2 days.

1.   What questions would you ask him?

Additional information: he reports a fever and malaise for the past day but no other GCA symptoms, and no previous episodes or past ocular history. The pain is lancinating and burning on the forehead and around the eye with eye ache and sensitivity to light. The eye exam is normal. Four days later, he returns with the appearance shown in the photo.

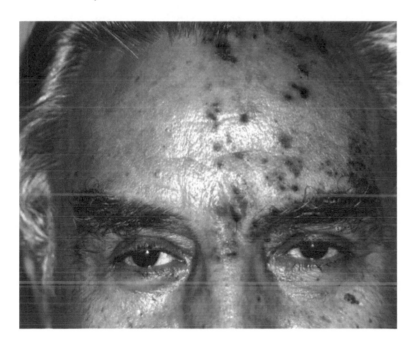

2.   What is the diagnosis?

3.   What does a lesion on the tip of the nose mean?

4.   What anterior segment eye findings would you look for?

5.   How would you treat this patient?

6.   If this patient was 37 years old, what additional history and testing would you obtain?

7.   What are the possible complications?

8.   What are the risk factors for PHN?

9.   How can this complication be treated?

1. Has he experienced any other related symptoms or any neurologic symptoms? It is important to ask specifically about symptoms of GCA: scalp tenderness (does it hurt when you brush your hair?), jaw claudication (does it hurt to chew food?), headaches, fever, unexpected weight loss, and joint pain (PMR). Has he had any previous episodes of eye pain and blurry vision? Did he experience loss of vision or just blurry vision? Is the blurry vision constant or intermittent? Was the onset sudden or gradual? Is there any redness or discharge? Characterize the pain (sharp, dull, pressure, radiation, superficial, deep, constant, intermittent, duration, severity, etc.). Does he have any past ocular history?

2. HZO or shingles caused by VZV.

3. Hutchinson sign, which is a strong indicator of ocular involvement (nasociliary branch of the ophthalmic nerve [CN V_1]).

4. Conjunctivitis, keratitis (epithelial, stromal, or endothelial), iritis, and increased IOP.

5. A 7-day course of an oral antiviral starting within 72 hours of the rash reduces the time course and risk and severity of ocular involvement. Famciclovir or valacyclovir is preferable to acyclovir because of reduced risk of PHN. Oral steroids also reduce the time course, duration and severity of acute pain, and the risk of PHN. Topical steroids and cycloplegic for iritis, and monitor IOP; may require low-dose topical steroid indefinitely to prevent recurrence of uveitis. If corneal epithelial involvement occurs, then add a topical antibiotic. Prevention of herpes zoster is with vaccination in patients aged ≥50 years (reduces incidence, severity, and duration of zoster, reduces incidence of pain, and reduces incidence of PHN).

6. Herpes zoster is rare in individuals <40 years old unless they are immunocompromised; therefore, a history of immunosuppression (cancer, HIV, etc.) should be determined and an HIV test considered.

7. Lid scarring (lagophthalmos, ectropion, entropion, trichiasis, madarosis), canalicular and punctal stenosis, symblepharon, exposure keratopathy, neurotrophic keratopathy, corneal scarring, scleritis, glaucoma, uveitis, iris atrophy and necrosis, cataract, CME, optic neuropathy, retinitis, cranial nerve palsies, orbital apex syndrome, and PHN.

8. Increasing age, severity of pain, severity of skin rash, presence of ocular involvement.

9. A variety of medications can be used to treat PHN including opioids, tricyclic antidepressants, gabapentin/pregabalin, cimetidine, carbamazepine, steroids, topical analgesics (lidocaine cream/gel, lidoderm patch, capsaicin cream), diphenhydramine (Benadryl), nerve blocks, and Botox injections.

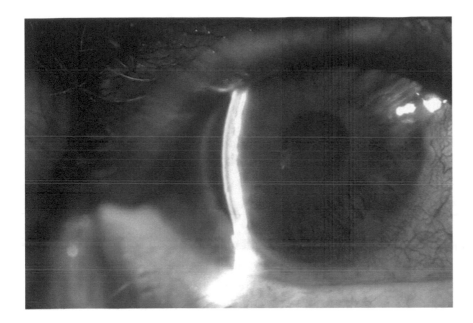

A 51-year-old woman woke up with decreased vision and eye pain in the right eye. It is hard for her to open her eyes for the exam, and she says she feels nauseous. She is allergic to penicillin and sulfa. The appearance of the anterior segment is shown in the photo.

1. What is the diagnosis?
2. What are the associations?
3. What exam findings would you expect to see?
4. How do you distinguish between appositional and synechial angle closure?
5. What is the mechanism of primary angle closure?
6. How would you treat this patient?

1. Acute angle-closure glaucoma.

2. Anatomic features that predispose to angle closure are small anterior segment (hyperopia, nanophthalmos, microcornea, microphthalmos), anterior iris insertion (Eskimos, Asians), and shallow anterior chamber (large lens, plateau iris configuration, loose or subluxed lens, pseudoexfoliation syndrome).

3. Decreased vision, mid-dilated poorly reactive pupil with possible RAPD, conjunctival injection, corneal epithelial edema, markedly elevated IOP, shallow anterior chamber, closed angle, iris bombe, and possibly mild anterior chamber cells and flare, peripheral anterior synechiae, iris atrophy, glaukomflecken, optic nerve swelling and hyperemia.

4. Indentation gonioscopy with a 4- or 6-mirror lens (ie, Zeiss, Posner, Sussman). Indenting the cornea forces aqueous fluid peripherally toward the angle. The angle opens if closure is appositional and remains closed if closure is synechial.

5. *Pupillary block*: acute lens–iris apposition causes aqueous to be sequestered in the posterior chamber, anterior bowing of the iris, and occlusion of the trabecular meshwork.

    Lens-induced iridotrabecular contact: the size of the crystalline lens is relatively too large, which causes iridocorneal angle narrowing and intermittent/chronic iridotrabecular contact. Chronic microtrauma causes posterior anterior synechaie and/or decreased aqueous outflow due to trabecular meshwork dysfunction resulting in increased IOP and eventual glaucomatous optic neuropathy.

6. Acute angle closure is an ophthalmic emergency that requires immediate lowering of IOP. Treatment is with multiple topical hypotensive drops (ie, β-blocker, α_2-agonist, carbonic anhydrase inhibitor [CAI], pilocarpine [may not be effective if IOP is > 40 mmHg owing to sphincter ischemia and may cause the lens–iris diaphragm to move forward, worsening pupillary block]) and oral agents (CAI and hyperosmotic agent, such as isosorbide, glycerin [contraindicated in diabetics], or IV mannitol [risk of cardiovascular adverse effects]). CAIs should not be used in this patient because of her sulfa allergy. Also, a topical steroid is added for inflammation. Laser peripheral iridotomy is the definitive treatment and performed when the cornea is clear enough to provide an adequate view. Topical glycerin may be necessary to clear corneal edema. A surgical iridectomy or cataract surgery may be necessary if a laser iridotomy cannot be performed.

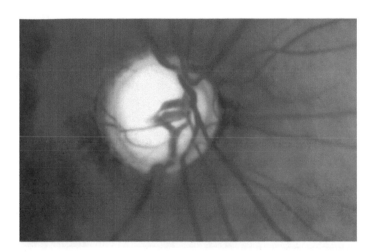

A 38-year-old man comes in for a complete eye exam. He says his vision has always been good, and his last exam was more than 10 years ago. Exam shows 20/20 vision in both eyes, a peripheral posterior cortical/subcapsular cataract, and optic cupping in the right eye.

1. What additional history would be helpful?
2. How would you work up this patient?

Additional information: the patient says he was hit with a tennis ball in the right eye as a child and had blurry vision for a week or two but was not hospitalized and had no eye surgery. He denies any steroid use. IOP is 34 mmHg OD with normal corneal pachymetry. There is an inferior arcuate scotoma on HVF testing. Gonioscopy of the angle shows:

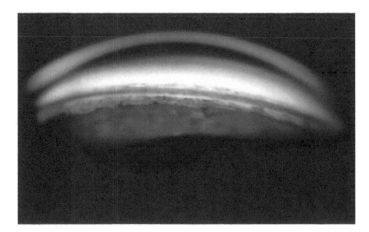

3. What finding is present?
4. What is the diagnosis?
5. What treatment would you recommend?
6. What surgical options are best for this type of glaucoma?

1. What is his past medical and ocular history? Is there a history of trauma, surgery, or steroid use? Does he take any medication? Does he have a family history of eye disease?

2. Slit-lamp exam with attention to signs of anterior segment injury (corneal scars, iris and angle tears, phacodonesis, cataract), check IOP, corneal pachymetry, gonioscopy, visual fields, optic nerve head photos, and nerve fiber layer analysis (OCT, confocal scanning laser ophthalmoscopy [Heidelberg retina tomograph], scanning laser polarimetry [GDx]).

3. Angle recession, which is a tear in the ciliary body between the longitudinal and circular fibers of the ciliary muscle.

4. Angle recession glaucoma.

5. Initial treatment with topical medications. Laser trabeculoplasty has a poor effect on angle recession, so surgery is usually considered as the next step.

6. Trabeculectomy with antimetabolite or glaucoma drainage implant.

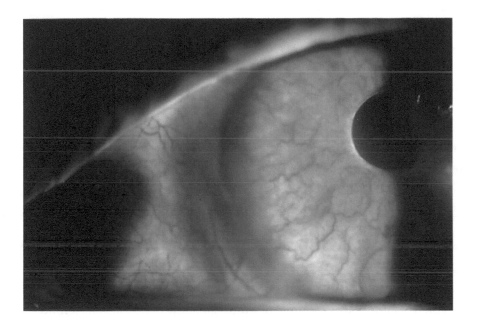

A 63-year-old man presents with decreased vision in the right eye.

1. What is the diagnosis?
2. What is the etiology?
3. What other findings would you look for on exam?
4. What is the treatment?
5. What are the complications of rubeosis?
6. What is the mechanism and treatment of NVG?

1. Rubeosis (iris neovascularization).

2. Ocular ischemia, most commonly due to PDR, central retinal vein occlusion, and carotid occlusive disease. Rubeosis is also associated with anterior segment ischemia, chronic retinal detachment, tumors, sickle cell retinopathy, and chronic inflammation.

3. RAPD, increased IOP, corneal edema, angle neovascularization, retinal neovascularization/hemorrhages, or optic nerve cupping. FA may demonstrate retinal nonperfusion and neovascularization. Iris angiogram will reveal neovascularization. Visual field testing may show glaucomatous defects.

4. Intravitreal anti-VEGF injection to acutely reduce the neovascularization, but eventually panretinal laser photocoagulation for retinal ischemia is needed for a more permanent treatment. Treatment of increased IOP or glaucoma may be necessary.

5. NVG and hyphema. If the underlying cause is PDR, then vitreous hemorrhage and traction retinal detachment can occur.

6. NVG is a form of secondary angle-closure glaucoma. Neovascularization of the iris and angle results in occlusion of the trabecular meshwork. NVG usually requires a glaucoma drainage implant or cyclodestructive procedure to adequately control IOP. Panretinal photocoagulation should also be applied.

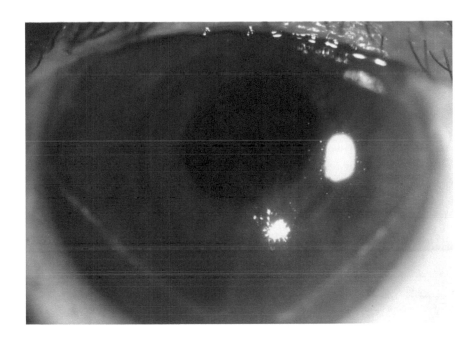

An 80-year-old woman reports blurry vision and pain in her right eye for several months. Her past ocular history is significant for cataract surgery 20 years ago.

1. What is the diagnosis?

2. What are the other causes of bullous keratopathy?

3. How would you treat her?

1. PBK due to a rigid anterior chamber IOL.

2. Corneal edema causing bullous keratopathy can also be due to aphakia, vitreocorneal touch, iridocorneal touch, severe or chronic keratitis, and breaks in Descemet membrane (ie, birth trauma).

3. Temporary treatment of the corneal edema and any inflammation is with topical steroids and a cycloplegic. If the patient develops ruptured bullae, she should be treated with a topical antibiotic, lubrication, and bandage contact lens. Amniotic membrane or a tarsorrhaphy may be necessary to heal a persistent epithelial defect. Anterior stromal puncture may help, but the bullae often recur. Definitive treatment is IOL explantation or exchange, and corneal transplantation may also be required (endothelial or penetrating keratoplasty). Consider a Gundersen flap for comfort in patients with poor visual potential or who cannot undergo surgery.

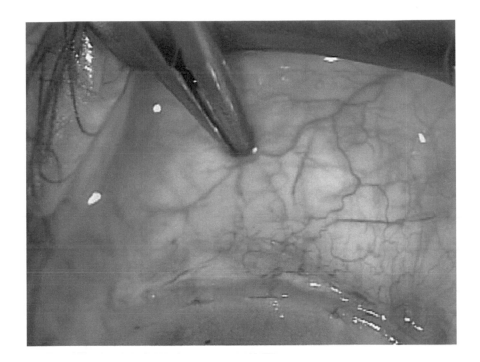

A 57-year-old woman with advanced glaucoma had a trabeculectomy last week. The appearance of her eye is shown.

1. What is the problem?
2. What findings would you look for on exam?
3. What is the differential diagnosis?
4. How does the anterior chamber appearance differ in angle-closure and malignant glaucoma?
5. You determine this patient has malignant glaucoma. How would you treat her?

1. Flat bleb.

2. IOP (decreased or increased), Seidel test, anterior chamber depth, and fundus appearance.

3. The differential diagnosis of a flat bleb depends on the IOP. If the IOP is low, then the cause is a bleb leak or choroidal detachment. If the IOP is high, then the cause is a suprachoroidal hemorrhage, pupillary block, or malignant glaucoma.

4. In angle closure, the anterior chamber is deeper centrally than peripherally, whereas in malignant glaucoma the entire anterior chamber is shallow.

5. Medical management is with a topical cycloplegic and aqueous suppressants. If this does not resolve the condition, then Nd:YAG laser anterior vitreolysis (for pseudophakic or aphakic eyes) or vitrectomy (for phakic eyes) may be required.

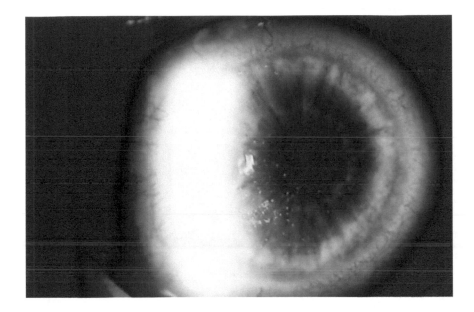

A 29-year-old man complains of worsening right eye pain and blurred vision for the last week. He reports several similar episodes in the past, but they all resolved within a few days. His past medical history is negative and he takes no medication.

1. What is the most likely diagnosis?
2. What other anterior segment signs you might find on exam?

Additional information: the patient has iris heterochromia and fine KP.

3. What is the diagnosis?
4. What are the eye findings specific to this form of anterior uveitis?
5. What is the etiology of iris heterochromia?
6. What is the treatment?

1. Iritis.

2. Ciliary injection, KP, anterior chamber cells and flare, posterior synechiae, altered IOP, iris atrophy, band keratopathy, cataract, cystoid macular edema.

3. Fuchs heterochromic iridocyclitis.

4. Iris heterochromia (lighter in affected eye), diffuse iris atrophy, small white stellate KP, fine-angle vessels (may bleed during gonioscopy, cataract surgery, or paracentesis), no synechiae, and minimal anterior chamber reaction.

5. The etiology depends on whether the condition is congenital or acquired and the involved iris is lighter (hypochromic) or darker (hyperchromic):

   Congenital:

   > **Hypochromic:** congenital Horner syndrome, Waardenburg syndrome, Hirschsprung disease, Parry–Romberg hemifacial atrophy.

   > **Hyperchromic:** ocular or oculodermal melanocytosis, iris pigment epithelium hamartoma.

   Acquired:

   > **Hypochromic:** acquired Horner syndrome, juvenile xanthogranuloma, iris metastatic carcinoma, Fuchs heterochromic iridocyclitis, stromal atrophy (glaucoma or inflammation).

   > **Hyperchromic:** siderosis, hemosiderosis, chalcosis, medication (topical prostaglandin analogs for glaucoma), iris nevus or melanoma, ICE syndrome, iris neovascularization.

6. Topical cycloplegic and steroids (typically there is a poor response to topical steroids, so they should not be used for long-term treatment), and may require treatment of elevated IOP.

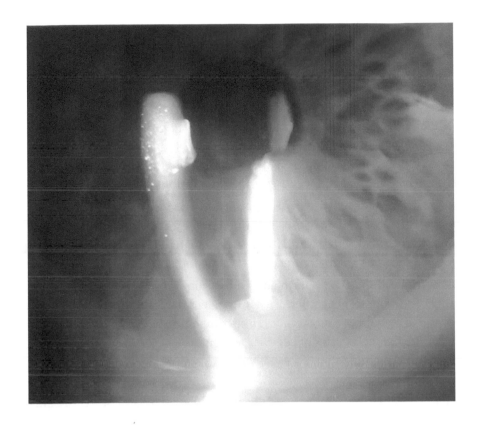

A 74-year-old woman undergoes complicated cataract surgery with posterior capsular rupture and retained lens fragment. On postoperative day 1, visual acuity is 20/60, there is mild conjunctival injection, moderate corneal edema, 2+ anterior chamber cells and flare, and a well-centered IOL in the sulcus.

1. How would you manage this patient?
2. What are the intraoperative signs of posterior capsular tear/rupture?
3. What surgical steps should be performed if a posterior capsular tear/rupture occurs?

1. The patient must be informed about the surgical complication, potential sequelae, and treatment plan. A dilated fundus exam is performed to identify retained lens material in the posterior segment and to examine the peripheral retina for tears or retinal detachment (increased risk with vitreous loss).

   Management of retained material after cataract surgery depends upon the size, type (cortical versus nuclear), and location (anterior segment versus posterior segment) of the lens fragment(s). Nuclear material, even small chips, are generally poorly tolerated and should be removed promptly because they can induce severe intraocular inflammation with elevated IOP, corneal edema, and CME. Small pieces of cortex can be observed and may resorb over weeks to months with topical steroid treatment and careful observation. Cortex sequestered in the capsular bag rarely causes any complications.

   The inflammation is treated with topical steroids and usually a topical NSAID as well, and the patient may require treatment for elevated IOP. If a piece of nucleus is identified in the anterior chamber, surgical extraction by an anterior segment surgeon is indicated. Similarly, if nuclear material is present in the vitreous cavity, the patient should be referred to a retinal surgeon for evaluation and removal.

2. The signs depend upon when this complication occurs. During hydrodissection or phacoemulsification, there is usually a sudden deepening of the anterior chamber. The lens nucleus may shift or tilt or even dislocate into the posterior segment. Further phacoemulsification is accompanied by poor followability when vitreous is present in the anterior chamber. Posterior capsular tear/rupture occurring during subsequent steps (ie, I/A, lens insertion or manipulation) is usually directly visible as sudden posterior capsule striae followed by a hole or split in the capsule.

3. It is important to prevent collapse of the anterior chamber since this causes the vitreous to move forward and usually results in rupture of the anterior vitreous face. Therefore, before removing an instrument from the main incision (ie, phaco or I/A tip), continue irrigation while injecting a dispersive OVD through a side port incision to maintain the space and sequester any remaining nuclear material in the anterior chamber. A Sheets glide can be inserted to prevent nuclear material from falling posteriorly. Any vitreous prolapsing forward must be removed by performing a thorough anterior vitrectomy. Triamcinolone (Kenalog or Triesence) can be used to help visualize vitreous strands in the anterior chamber. The remaining nuclear pieces can be removed manually or with low-flow phaco settings (ie, lower the irrigation bottle height, reduce the aspiration flow rate and vacuum), and then the remaining cortex can be removed manually, with an I/A probe, or with a vitrector. Finally, an IOL is inserted in an appropriate location, and its stability is checked to make sure it is secure. Depending on the type and position of the IOL, prior or after its insertion Miochol or Miostat can be injected to constrict the pupil. If the pupil does not become small and round, then vitreous may be prolapsing through the pupil or the IOL may be causing pupil ovalization or iris tuck, so additional manipulations may be required.

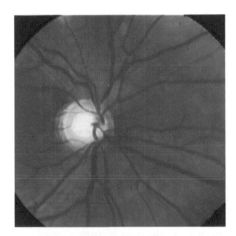

A 55-year-old man is found to have generous optic cups on routine eye exam.

1. What is the differential diagnosis?
2. What other history and exam findings are relevant?

Additional information: the patient is a low myope with no past ocular history. He denies previous trauma or steroid use, and there is no family history of glaucoma. His vision is 20/20 and the IOP is 18 mmHg OU, anterior segment exam is normal except for trace cortical changes in the crystalline lens OU, and posterior segment exam shows large optic cups OU.

3. What testing would you perform?

Additional information: on subsequent exam, the IOP is 19 mmHg and corneal pachymetry measures 540 microns OU. There is a small hemorrhage present at the inferior disc margin OS. Humphrey visual field testing shows an enlarged blindspot OD and a small superior nasal step OS.

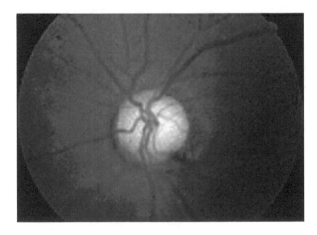

4. What is the diagnosis?
5. How would you manage this patient?

1. Physiologic cupping (usually myopic individuals), POAG; with large diurnal variations, "burned-out" secondary open-angle glaucoma (ie, pigmentary, uveitic, traumatic, steroid-induced glaucomas), chronic angle closure, NTG, neurologic disease (optic neuropathy, optic neuritis, chiasmal compressive lesions; usually have more pallor than cupping).

2. History of trauma, steroid use, uveitis, elevated IOP, family history of glaucoma, myopia. Exam findings suggestive of glaucomatous optic nerve damage in such a patient include Krukenburg spindle, keratic precipitates, iris transillumination defects, narrow angles, iris or angle tears, synechiae (peripheral anterior or posterior), elevated IOP, phacodonesis, PSC or traumatic cataract, nerve fiber layer defects, asymmetric cupping, splinter hemorrhage at nerve head.

3. Tonometry, corneal pachymetry, gonioscopy, visual fields, optic nerve head photos, and nerve fiber layer analysis; also consider performing a diurnal curve, optic nerve blood flow measurement (color Doppler imaging, laser Doppler flowmetry), ERG, VEP, and neurologic workup. Obtaining old ophthalmic records, if available, can be helpful.

4. NTG.

5. Treatment is to reduce IOP with medication, laser, or surgery. The CNTGS demonstrated that lowering IOP by 30% or more reduced the rate of visual field loss; however, rate of progression without treatment is variable and usually slow (half of untreated patients had no progression after 5 years). NTG is more difficult to treat than POAG.

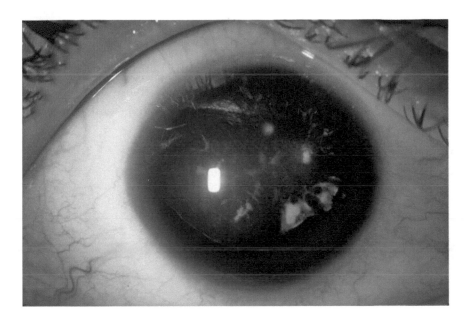

A 31-year-old man is noted to have ocular abnormalities on undilated slit-lamp exam.

1. What findings are shown in the photo, and what is the diagnosis?
2. What is the etiology?
3. What are the associated findings?
4. What is the treatment?

1. Absence of iris and cataract; aniridia.

2. Aniridia is a rare, congenital defect in which the iris is absent bilaterally except for a small peripheral remnant. The defect is hereditary or sporadic and has been mapped to chromosome 11p13 (*PAX6* gene).

3. Aniridia causes photophobia and glare; findings include decreased vision, nystagmus, strabismus, and amblyopia. It is associated with lens opacities (up to 80%), glaucoma (up to 50%), ectopia lentis, corneal pannus, optic nerve, and foveal hypoplasia. There are three types of aniridia:

   AN 1: most common (85%), autosomal dominant, only ocular findings.

   AN 2: 13%, sporadic, associated with Wilms tumor (Miller syndrome and WAGR syndrome).

   AN 3: 2%, autosomal recessive, associated with mental retardation and cerebellar ataxia (Gillespie syndrome) but not Wilms tumor.

4. Treatment for photophobia and glare is a cosmetic/painted contact lens. An artificial iris implant can be inserted at the time of cataract surgery. Patients may require treatment for increased IOP and glaucoma.

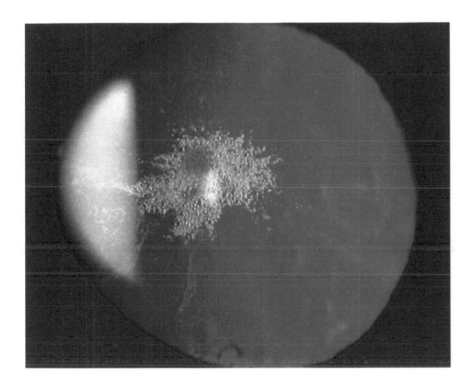

A 48-year-old man complains of blurry vision in his right eye. His BCVA is 20/80 OD (with minimal improvement with pinhole) and 20/20 OS. Besides the finding shown in the photo, his eye exam is otherwise normal.

1. What is the diagnosis?
2. What are the causes and typical symptoms of this type of cataract?
3. What are the indications for cataract surgery?
4. Does this patient have any increased risk of complications from cataract surgery?

1. PSC.

2. PSCs are associated with aging, steroids, trauma, ionizing radiation, intraocular inflammation, diabetes, high myopia, retinitis pigmentosa, Refsum disease, and atopic dermatitis. The characteristic symptoms are photophobia and glare especially from bright lights (ie, headlights while driving at night) and variable decreased vision typically worse at near than distance. Other symptoms of cataracts are reduced contrast and color sensitivity and sometimes monocular diplopia or polyopia.

3. The indication for cataract surgery is when the patient desires improved vision because of visual symptoms interfering with daily activities. Rarely, cataract surgery is performed for medical reasons such as the cataract is causing glaucoma or uveitis, or the cataract is interfering with the examination or treatment of another ocular disease (ie, macular degeneration, diabetic retinopathy, glaucoma) because the posterior segment cannot be adequately evaluated through the lens opacity.

4. There is no increased risk of a surgical complication unless the cataract is associated with trauma that has resulted in other ocular problems (ie, zonular weakness or dehiscence, vitreous prolapse, corneal scarring interfering with visualization of the lens).

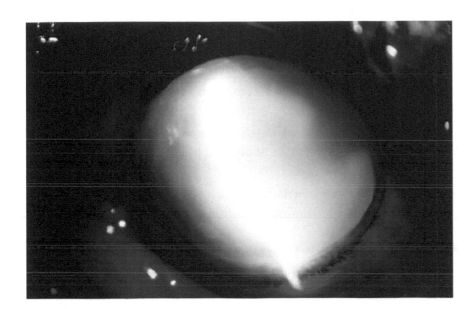

An 87-year-old woman is seen urgently for increasing eye pain and loss of vision for several days.

1. What does the photo show?
2. What is the differential diagnosis?
3. What are the characteristics of each?

Additional information: exam shows visual acuity of LP only, the IOP is 27 mmHg, the anterior chamber is deep, and there is a 3+ anterior chamber reaction with white flocculent material.

4. What is the treatment?

1. Mature cataract and conjunctival injection. The anterior chamber (depth and presence of inflammation) cannot be assessed from the photo.

2. Lens-induced glaucoma: phacolytic, phacomorphic, or lens particle.

3. *Phacolytic*: hypermature cataract leaks lens proteins through an intact capsule; trabecular meshwork obstructed by lens proteins and macrophages that ingest them.

    Phacomorphic: enlarged cataractous lens pushes the iris forward; the trabecular meshwork is obstructed by the iris (secondary angle closure). Risk factors include hyperopia, short axial length, and shallow anterior chamber depth.

    Lens particle: lens material from penetrating trauma or retained after cataract surgery causes inflammation (more than phacolytic and higher IOP, synechiae and inflammatory membranes); trabecular meshwork obstructed by lens material.

4. Topical treatment for inflammation (steroid and cycloplegic) and increased intraocular pressure should be initiated promptly. The definitive treatment for phacolytic glaucoma is urgent cataract surgery.

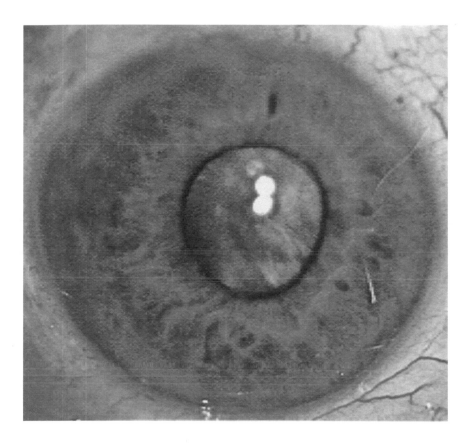

A 78-year-old man reports a gradual decrease in vision. On exam, his visual acuity is 20/60 OD and 20/80 OS. Fundus exam is normal OU.

1. What significant findings are apparent in the post-dilation slit-lamp photo?
2. What history would be helpful?

Additional information: his ocular history is negative except for myopia, he denies any eye trauma, inflammation, or surgery. He has difficulty with urination and has been treated with tamsulosin (Flomax) for 6 years.

3. What condition may occur during cataract surgery, and what risks does this pose?
4. How is this condition managed?

1. Cataract and poor pupillary dilation.

2. What is his past ocular, medical, and medication history? Has he had any ocular trauma, surgery, or been treated for any eye problems? Does he have an enlarged prostate or high blood pressure? What medications has he taken?

3. IFIS is a condition caused by α-1A adrenergic receptor antagonists, most commonly and severely by tamsulosin. IFIS is characterized by a variable degree of poor pupillary dilation, and floppy/atonic iris that billows, prolapses, and becomes miotic during surgery. This increases the risk of posterior capsular rupture, zonular dehiscence, vitreous loss, retained lens fragments, alternate lens placement, iris damage, and misshapen pupil.

4. Mild forms may respond to preoperative topical atropine and intraocular preservative-free epinephrine. More severe forms require iris stabilization with one or more of the following: dispersive/viscoadaptive OVDs (eg, Healon 5, Arshinoff soft-shell and ultimate soft-shell technique), pupil expanders (eg, Malyugin ring, Graether ring, I-ring), iris hooks, and low-flow fluidics during phacoemulsification. Manual stretching (ie, with microhooks as used to enlarge small pupils due to iris fibrosis or adhesions) is ineffective with an atonic iris and should be avoided.

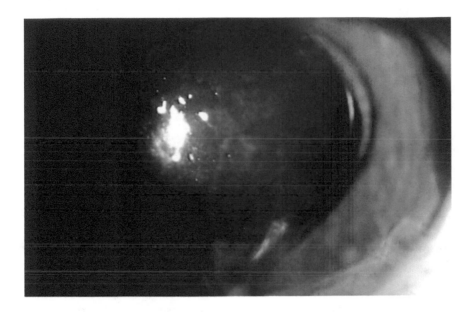

A 70-year-old woman notices blurry vision and photophobia on postoperative day 1 following cataract surgery.

1. What finding is present?
2. What is the differential diagnosis?
3. What other history is helpful?

Additional information: she has no history of corneal endothelial dystrophy. Cataract surgery was routine and uncomplicated. She reports mild discomfort and denies any floaters. On exam, her visual acuity is 20/100, IOP is 12 mmHg, conjunctiva is mildly injected, anterior chamber is deep with 2+ cells and 4+ flare and no vitreous prolapse, IOL is well centered, posterior capsule is intact, and anterior vitreous is clear.

4. What is the diagnosis?
5. What are the characteristics of this condition?
6. What is the etiology?
7. How is TASS treated?
8. What are the possible complications?

1. Corneal edema.

2. Corneal edema only, acute postoperative endophthalmitis, TASS, retained lens material.

3. Were there any intraoperative complications? Was an unusually high level of phaco energy used? Was there obvious corneal edema present at the end of surgery? Did she have significant cornea guttata preoperatively? Does she have any pain or floaters?

4. TASS.

5. TASS is a sterile postoperative inflammation of the anterior segment. It usually presents within 12–48 hours after surgery (most commonly cataract) and may be mild or severe. Characteristic findings include decreased visual acuity, diffuse corneal edema, fibrin in the anterior chamber (may have hypopyon), normal or high IOP, and minimal or no vitritis. There is typically less redness, pain, and anterior chamber reaction than in endophthalmitis.

6. TASS is caused by contaminants from surgical instruments, intraocular solutions, or IOL implant. These include particulate matter, bacterial endotoxins, denatured OVD, imbalanced solutions, enzymes, detergents, medications, and preservatives.

7. Frequent topical steroids (up to every hour and consider oral steroid in severe cases), consider topical NSAID, and may require ocular hypotensive medications if the IOP becomes elevated. In severe or delayed cases, treat with topical antibiotic and perform aqueous and vitreous taps for culture to rule out infectious endophthalmitis (usually presents 4–7 days after surgery).

8. Severe inflammation can cause intraocular damage, particularly to the corneal endothelium, trabecular meshwork, iris, and macula resulting in corneal edema, glaucoma, iris atrophy, and macular edema, respectively. Endothelial keratoplasty for corneal decompensation should be delayed for at least 3 months in order to prevent graft failure.

A 43-year-old woman comes in for an annual eye exam and is found to have shallow anterior chambers and narrow angles on gonioscopy. She is asymptomatic, her vision is 20/20 OU, and the rest of the exam is normal. After prophylactic laser iridotomies, her IOP is 17 mmHg OU, the iridotomies are patent, and gonioscopy reveals narrow angles.

1. What test would you order?

Additional information: UBM shows:

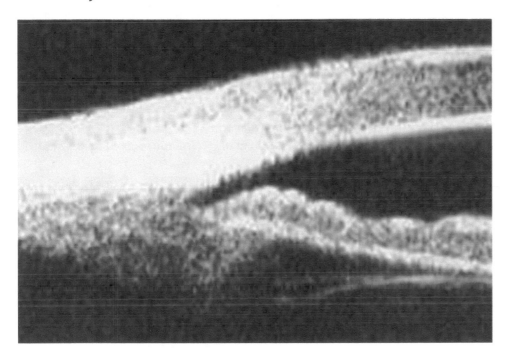

2. What is the diagnosis?
3. What is the pathophysiology of this condition?
4. How would you manage this?
5. What are the etiologies of secondary angle closure?

1. UBM.

2. Plateau iris syndrome.

3. Plateau iris is characterized by anteriorly rotated ciliary processes, which push the peripheral iris forward resulting in a deep chamber centrally and flat iris contour with a sharp dropoff peripherally. Dilation causes the peripheral iris to fold into the angle and occlude the trabecular meshwork. There is no pupillary block.

4. Laser iridoplasty and miotics.

5. *With pupillary block*: lens-induced (phacomorphic, dislocated lens, microspherophakia), seclusio pupillae, aphakic or pseudophakic pupillary block, silicone oil, nanophthalmos.

   Without pupillary block:

   Posterior "pushing" mechanism (mechanical or anterior displacement of the lens–iris diaphragm): plateau iris syndrome, inflammation (scleritis, uveitis, panretinal photocoagulation), congestion (scleral buckle, nanophthalmos), choroidal effusion (hypotony, uveal effusion, medication), suprachoroidal hemorrhage, aqueous misdirection (malignant glaucoma), posterior segment pressure (tumor, expansile gas, exudative retinal detachment), developmental abnormalities (persistent hyperplastic primary vitreous, retinopathy of prematurity).

   Anterior "pulling" mechanism (adherence of iris to the trabecular meshwork or membranes over the trabecular meshwork): epithelial (downgrowth or ingrowth), endothelial (ICE syndrome, PPCD), neovascular, postinflammatory PAS, adhesion from trauma, mesodermal dysgenesis syndromes.

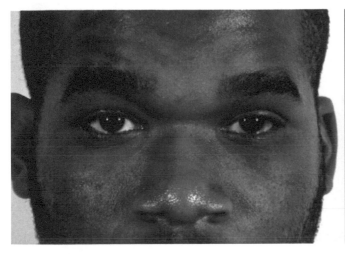 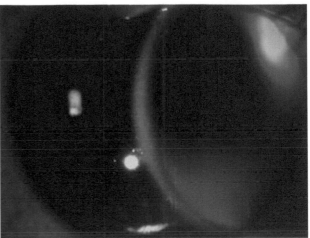

A 39-year-old man presents after being punched in the left eye. He complains of blurry vision and pain.

1. What is the diagnosis?

2. What is the treatment?

3. What is an 8-ball hyphema?

4. What are the indications for anterior chamber washout?

1. Hyphema.

2. Topical steroids and cycloplegic, may require treatment of increased IOP (do not use miotic agents or prostaglandin analogs, and avoid carbonic anhydrase inhibitors in patients with sickle cell disease), consider aminocaproic acid. Daily observation for the first 5 days to monitor the IOP and check for a rebleed. The patient should avoid aspirin-containing products, remain at bedrest, sleep with the head of the bed elevated, and protect the eye with a shield. Anterior chamber washout may be required.

3. A hyphema that has clotted and appears black or purple owing to impaired aqueous circulation and deoxygenated blood, which prevents resorption.

4. Anterior chamber washout is performed for corneal bloodstaining, uncontrolled elevated IOP, persistent blood clot, and rebleed.

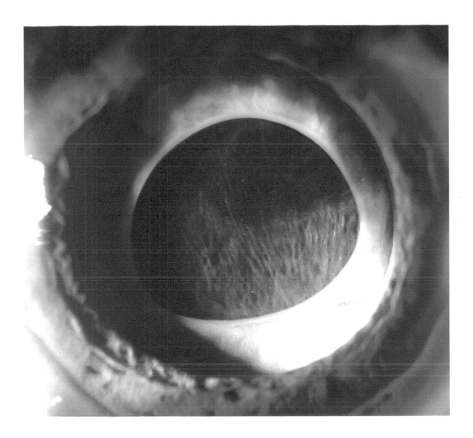

A 68-year-old man complains of fuzzy vision 2 years after cataract surgery.

1. What does the photo show?

2. What are the risk factors?

3. What is the etiology?

4. What are the indications for Nd:YAG laser treatment?

5. What are the potential complications of laser posterior capsulotomy?

1. PCO and anterior capsular phimosis (anterior capsular contraction syndrome).

2. *PCO:* younger age, uveitis, IOL material (silicone > acrylic) and edge design (round > square), incomplete cortical cleanup.

   Phimosis: small capsulorhexis, zonular weakness, pseudoexfoliation syndrome, uveitis, retinitis pigmentosa, diabetes, IOL material (silicone) and type (plate haptic).

3. Epithelial cell proliferation (Elschnig pearls) and fibrosis of the capsule.

4. PCO (posterior capsulotomy, selective capsulotomies for Crystalens vaulting problems), phimosis (radial anterior capsulotomies), capsular block syndrome (anterior or posterior capsulotomy).

5. The risks are small but include increased IOP; iritis; IOL optic damage; IOL dislocation; posterior vitreous detachment; cystoid macular edema; corneal, iris, or retinal burns; retinal tear and detachment; and hyphema.

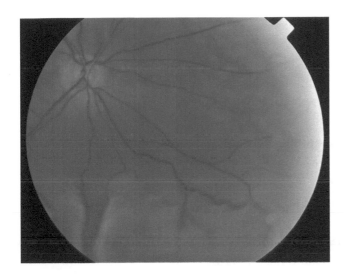

A 47-year-old woman reports blurry vision for several weeks.

1. What does the photo show?
2. What are the possible etiologies?
3. What other exam findings would you look for?
4. What other tests would be helpful and why?

Additional information: an ultrasound evaluation is performed. The B-scan reveals a mass, and the A-scan shows:

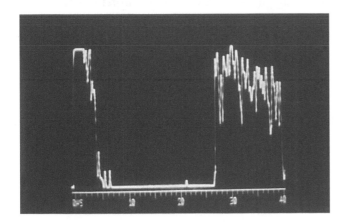

5. What is the most likely diagnosis and why?
6. How would you treat the patient?
7. What is the prognosis?

1. A dome-shaped, exudative RD without corrugation or surface membranes. In addition, there is no evidence of retinal traction. No obvious mass is seen in the picture.

2. The causes of an exudative RD include uveitis (VKH syndrome, sympathetic ophthalmia, pars planitis, posterior scleritis), tumors (especially retinal capillary hemangioma/von Hippel–Lindau disease, choroidal hemangioma, choroidal malignant melanoma), and hypertension. Other causes are glomerulonephritis, eclampsia/preeclampsia, hypothyroidism, Coats disease, scleritis, and CSC.

3. In general, exudative RDs are located inferiorly, display shifting fluid, and have a smooth, dome-shaped appearance. The appearance of a smooth, RD behind the lens is almost pathognomonic for exudative RD. Chronic exudative RD can lead to neovascular glaucoma.

    It is important to perform a careful depressed dilated fundus examination to evaluate for peripheral retinal horseshoe tears and holes to rule out a RRD, as well as evaluation for traction membranes to rule out a TRD. The fluid in RRD does not shift, and serous detachments do not develop PVR. TRDs are usually taut and immobile with a concave surface that does not extend to the ora serrata.

4. An FA is useful to evaluate for tumors (intrinsic vasculature, feeder vessels) and vascular abnormalities. ICG angiography is superior to FA to show intrinsic vascularity, hot spots, and washout phenomenon in tumors. A B-scan ultrasound should be performed to confirm the shifting fluid, evaluate choroidal thickness (uveal effusion syndrome), and, more importantly, to evaluate for masses. An A-scan ultrasound is used to evaluate internal reflectivity if a mass is found. OCT is useful to verify a thickened choroid using enhanced depth imaging techniques in uveitic and CSC conditions, image the subretinal fluid and/or cystoid macular edema. Although rarely necessary, orbital imaging can be performed.

5. Choroidal hemangioma because of the high internal reflectivity on A-scan.

6. The decision to treat is individualized based on the extent of symptoms, loss of vision, and potential for visual recovery. The aim of treatment is to induce tumor atrophy with resolution of subretinal fluid and tumor-induced foveal distortion without destroying the function of overlying retina. The goal is not to obliterate the tumor. Treatment options consist of laser photocoagulation (moderately intense, white reaction on the tumor surface to eliminate serous exudation), cryotherapy, ocular PDT with verteporfin (Visudyne) using standard treatment parameters, transpupillary thermotherapy, I-125 plaque brachytherapy, and low-dose external beam radiation therapy.

7. Visual loss can be progressive and irreversible when the fovea is involved in chronic cases. Poor visual acuity results can be expected despite resolution of fluid exudates from chronic macular edema and photoreceptor loss.

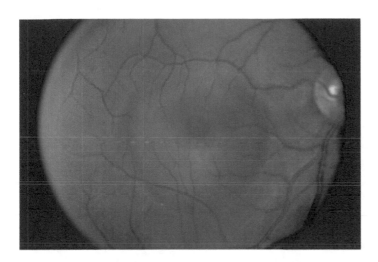

A 44-year-old man is worried about blurry vision in the right eye for the past 2 weeks.

1. What is the differential diagnosis?
2. What tests would be helpful?

Additional information: the FA shows:

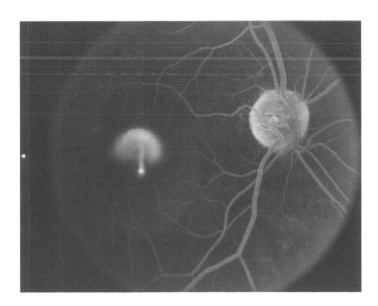

3. What is demonstrated, and what is the diagnosis?
4. How would you manage this patient?

1. CSC, inflammatory choroidal disorders (VKH syndrome), uveal effusion syndrome, optic nerve pit, choroidal tumor, vitelliform macular detachment, pigment epithelial detachment from other causes including CNV.

2. OCT to characterize the features present along with the obvious subretinal fluid including checking for macular schisis or optic nerve excavations seen with an optic nerve pit, a thickened choroid that is seen in VKH, CSC, and uveal effusion syndrome, or the characteristic OCT appearance of vitelliform lesions. An FA would be useful to rule out CNV (although rare in this age group) and to visualize the hyperfluorescence early with late pooling of a pigment epithelial detachment and the subretinal fluid. If both these tests fail to determine the diagnosis, ICG can show hyperfluorescence with late staining in CSC, vascularity with tumors, and rule out CNV. OCTA can be useful to also rule out CNV.

3. The FA shows "smoke-stack" leakage into the pigment epithelial detachment characteristic of CSC; however, this classic appearance is seen in only about 10% of cases.

4. Observation initially since most cases resolve spontaneously over 6 weeks. Discontinue any oral, topical, inhaled steroids. Off-label, anti-mineralocorticoid oral therapy (spironolactone or eplenerone), off-label rifampin, thermal laser treatment or verteporfin (Visudyne) ocular PDT can be considered for patients who require more rapid visual recovery because of occupational reasons, poor vision in the fellow eye due to CSC, no resolution of fluid after several months, recurrent episodes with poor vision, or in severe forms of CSC. Treatment reduces the duration of symptoms but does not affect the final visual acuity.

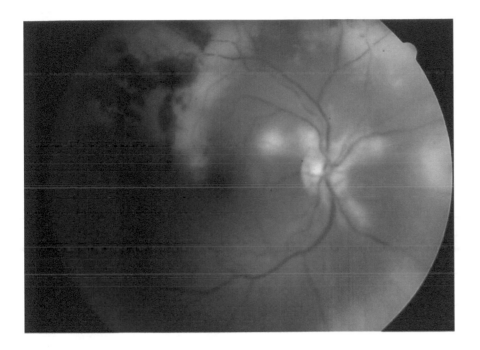

A 49-year-old man complains of acute eye pain with decreased vision and photophobia.

1. What does the photo demonstrate?
2. What is the differential diagnosis?
3. What other findings would you look for on exam?
4. What laboratory tests would be helpful?

Additional information: the anterior chamber PCR is positive for HSV, and the HIV test is negative.

5. What is the diagnosis?
6. What is the treatment?
7. What are the potential complications?

1. A well-defined area of retinal necrosis with retinal whitening and intraretinal hemorrhages.

2. ARN, PORN, syphilis, CMV retinitis, toxoplasmosis, sclopoteria, lymphoma, sarcoidosis, HORV; associated with intraocular vancomycin, and aminoglycoside toxicity.

3. Evidence of granulomatous anterior uveitis, vitritis, and retinal vasculitis.

4. PCR testing of intraocular fluid is the most precise method to determine the cause of the viral retinitis: VZV, HSV, or, rarely, CMV, or EBV. Alternatively, blood testing for VZV and HSV (type 1 and 2) immunoglobulin G and M (IgG and IgM) titers can be performed. The immune status should be obtained to verify whether the patient is immunocompetent because it is important to differentiate ARN from PORN, which occurs in immunocompromised patients with minimal inflammation and vasculitis.

5. ARN.

6. Immediately treat with antivirals since any delay in therapy can cause a dramatic increase in the retinitis. Typically, systemic acyclovir (IV until resolution of the retinitis, then oral for 1–2 months); alternatively, if the lesions are more peripheral, then use oral therapy with valacyclovir instead of IV therapy. Ganciclovir is an alternative. It is important to follow blood urea nitrogen and creatinine levels for nephrotoxicity. Both oral and topical steroids can be started after the patient begins to respond to prevent inflammatory complications. Also treat with intravitreal foscarnet, follow closely for signs of regression, and if none seen additional injections may be required.

7. Patients with ARN are at high risk of developing RRD with numerous holes and giant tears due to retinal necrosis. In addition, very careful observation of the fellow eye is important to rule out involvement.

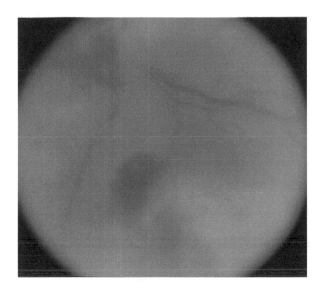

A 65-year-old man presents with blurred vision and floaters in both eyes for several months. On exam, his eyes are white and quiet, and there are bilateral dense sheets of vitreous cells. He says he has been treated by an outside doctor with topical steroids with no response.

1. What additional history would you want to know?
2. What is the differential diagnosis?
3. What tests would you perform?

Additional information: the pathology from a vitreous biopsy shows:

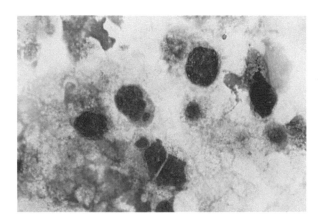

4. What is the diagnosis?
5. How would you treat this patient?
6. What additional testing should be performed?
7. What is the prognosis?

1. Has he had any unexplained fevers and chills, night sweats, fatigue, headaches, or weight loss? What is the past medical history, especially any cancer history? Is there any lymphadenopathy (especially cervical and supraclavicular), or any CNS symptoms?

2. Anything that produces a chronic vitritis including infectious and noninfectious uveitis such as birdshot chorioretinopathy, pars planitis, toxoplasmosis, syphilis, sarcoidosis, multifocal choroiditis, APMPPE, Behçets disease, tuberculosis, and ARN; however, for a patient in this age group with these signs, PIOL is of greatest concern.

3. Since PIOL is a masquerade syndrome, complete laboratory testing to rule out other uveitic entities should be done including CBC, ESR, ACE, lysozyme, HLA-B 27 and 51, ANA test, and VDRL or RPR, FTA-ABS or MHA-TP testing. For additional testing paradigm, see Case 142.

   With negative laboratory testing, a thorough neurologic evaluation should be performed in search of CNS involvement including MRI of the brain and lumbar puncture for CNS cytology. If both are negative, then a diagnostic pars plana vitrectomy should be performed. An undilute vitreous biopsy (approximately 1 cc) should be sent for cytology, flow cytometry analysis for B- and T-cell markers and kappa/lambda light chains. Other ancillary tests include the measurement of IL-6 and IL-10 (high IL-10 and high ratio of IL-10 to IL-6 are suggestive of intraocular lymphoma).

4. Diffuse large B-cell non-Hodgkin lymphoma.

5. The treatment of PVRL is still controversial and includes intravitreal methotrexate and/or rituximab, and orbital radiation in cases without any CNS involvement. However, the majority of patients do develop CNS involvement, so most oncologists treat with chemotherapy with blood–brain barrier disruption or high-dose systemic methotrexate.

6. A complete metastatic survey (imaging studies of the chest and abdomen) and bone marrow biopsy.

7. More than 67% will develop CNS lymphoma within a mean of 29 months. The prognosis is poor if there is brain involvement.

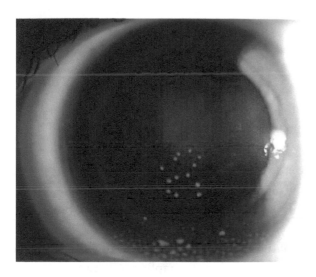

A 42-year-old woman reports pain, photophobia, redness, and decreased vision for 4 days. She recalls having had a similar episode several years ago.

1. What finding is shown, and what is the diagnosis?
2. What is the differential diagnosis?
3. What other findings may be present?
4. How would you work up a patient with granulomatous uveitis?

Additional Information: the appearance of her retina is shown.

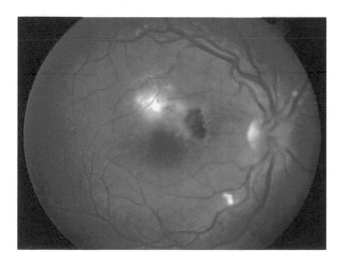

5. What is the diagnosis?
6. What is the treatment?

1. This patient has large mutton-fat KP, which is a sign of granulomatous uveitis.

2. Syphilis, tuberculosis, leprosy, brucellosis, toxoplasmosis, *Propionibacterium acnes* chronic endophthalmitis, fungal infection (*Cryptococcus*, *Aspergillus*), HIV, sarcoidosis, VKH syndrome, sympathetic ophthalmia, and a phacoanaphylactic reaction.

3. Ciliary injection, anterior chamber cells and flare, hypopyon, iris nodules, rubeosis, synechiae, increased or decreased IOP, cataract, pars planitis, optic nerve hyperemia, chorioretinitis, periphlebitis, and cystoid macular edema.

4. A basic battery of laboratory tests is recommended to determine the cause of granulomatous uveitis in a patient with a negative history, review of systems, and medical examination. This includes CBC with differential, ESR, VDRL or RPR (syphilis), FTA-ABS or MHA-TP (syphilis), ELISA or indirect IFA for toxoplasma IgM and IgG titers, ACE (sarcoidosis), lysozyme.

    Other laboratory tests can be ordered according to the patient's history including ANA, RF; juvenile idiopathic arthritis, ELISA for Lyme IgM and IgG, HIV antibody test, chest radiographs or CT scan (sarcoidosis, tuberculosis), sacroiliac radiographs (ankylosing spondylitis), and urinalysis.

    Special diagnostic laboratory tests can also be considered if the diagnosis is still unclear including HLA typing (HLA-A29: Birdshot chorioretinopathy), in the presence of vasculitis: ANCA (granulomatosis with polyarteritis, polyarteritis nodosa), Raji cell and C1q binding assays for circulating immune complexes (SLE, systemic vasculitides), complement proteins: C3, C4, total complement (SLE, cryoglobulinemia, glomerulonephritis), and soluble IL-2 receptor.

5. Toxoplasmosis chorioretinitis.

6. Topical steroids and cycloplegic are prescribed to treat the anterior inflammation. Systemic steroids are added for posterior pole lesions or those with intense inflammation.

    Small peripheral lesions may be observed since they often heal spontaneously, especially in immunocompetent individuals. If a patient has decreased vision, moderate to severe vitreous inflammation, or lesions that threaten the macula, papillomacular bundle, or optic nerve, he/she should be treated for 4–6 weeks with antibiotics that kill tachyzoites in the retina (note: they do not affect cysts). Most patients respond well to trimethoprim–sulfamethoxazole (Bactrim). For aggressive lesions or posterior pole lesions, triple therapy can be considered with pyrimethamine (Daraprim), folinic acid (leucovorin), and one of the following: sulfadiazine, clindamycin, clarithromycin, azithromycin, or atovaquone. Immunocompromised patients and high-risk patients may require prophylactic treatment.

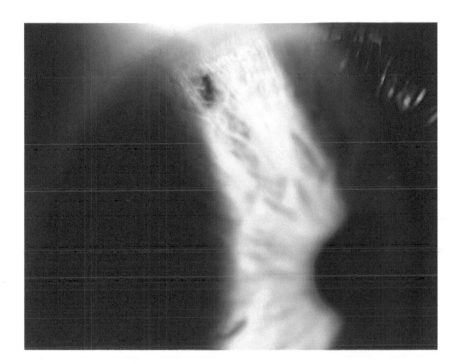

A 38-year-old man with no previous ocular history reports irritation of his right eye after doing some work around the house. On exam, the patient has 20/20 vision and normal intraocular pressure. The appearance of the anterior segment is shown above.

1. What abnormality is present, and what is the likely cause?

2. How would you work up this patient?

3. How are foreign bodies classified?

4. What findings are seen in chalcosis and siderosis?

5. What complication may occur, and what is the most common organism?

6. How would you treat this patient?

1. Iris defect due to an IOFB.

2. Ask a detailed history about the type of work he was performing (ie, hammering, sawing, power tools)? Did he wear eye protection? Did he feel something hit or poke his eye?

   Obtain an orbital CT or X-ray to identify any IOFB (not an MRI if a metallic IOFB is suspected).

3. *Inert*: do not require removal (ie, glass, plastic, sand, stone, ceramic, gold, platinum, silver, aluminum).

   Reactive: cause inflammation/toxicity and must be removed (ie, copper [≥ 85% causes severe endophthalmitis, <85% causes chalcosis, <70% is relatively inert], iron [siderosis], wood/plant material [significant inflammation and higher risk of traumatic endophthalmitis]).

4. *Chalcosis*: mild intraocular inflammation, deposition of copper in the anterior lens capsule (sunflower cataract) and Descemet membrane (Kayser–Fleischer ring), and retinal degeneration. The iris may become green and the pupil sluggishly reactive to light.

   Siderosis: iris heterochromia (hyperchromic on involved side), mid-dilated minimally reactive pupil, lens discoloration (brown-orange dots from iron deposition in lens epithelium, generalized yellowing from involvement of cortex), vitritis, pigmentary RPE degeneration with sclerosis of vessels, retinal thinning, and atrophy.

   In both conditions, the ERG is reduced or even absent.

5. Post-traumatic endophthalmitis, usually caused by *Staphylococcus*. The risk of infectious endophthalmitis (2%–7%) is higher with retained foreign body, delayed surgery (>24 hours), rural setting (soil contamination), and crystalline lens disruption.

6. Surgical exploration and repair with removal of any reactive foreign body material should be performed as soon as possible. The use of intravitreal (vancomycin [1 mg/0.1 mL], amikacin [0.4 mg/0.1 mL], or ceftazidime [2.25 mg/0.1 mL]) and systemic antibiotics (IV vancomycin 1 g q12h or cefazolin 1 g q8h; ceftazidime 1 g q12h) is usually performed to prevent endophthalmitis. In cases with wood or rural setting, also consider prophylaxis against fungal organisms.

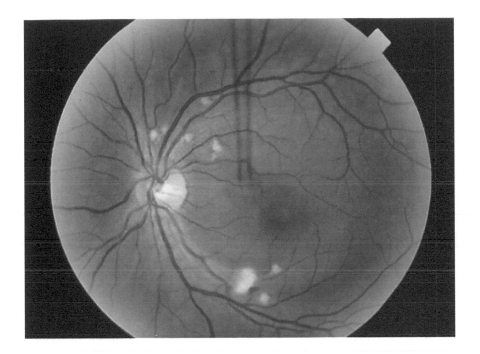

A 29-year-old man presents for a routine eye evaluation. His exam is normal except for the retinal exam.

1. What findings are depicted?
2. What is the differential diagnosis?
3. How would you work up this patient?

Additional information: the patient is HIV positive.

4. How would you treat him?

1. Multiple CWS, microaneurysms, and intraretinal hemorrhages.

2. The most common causes of CWS are diabetes and hypertension. Other causes include ischemic (RVO, ocular ischemic syndrome, severe anemia, preeclampsia, carotid artery obstruction), embolic (carotid emboli, cardiac emboli, deep venous emboli, white blood cell emboli [Purtscher retinopathy], severe chest compression/long bone fractures, foreign bodies [IV drug abuse], amniotic fluid embolization), infectious (HIV, Rocky Mountain Spotted Fever, cat-scratch fever [*Bartonella henselae*], toxoplasmosis, subacute bacterial endocarditis, leptospirosis, onchocerciasis [river blindness], fungemia), toxic (interferon, methotrexate), radiation induced, neoplastic (lymphoma, leukemia, metastatic carcinoma, Hodgkin disease), immune-mediated (SLE, sarcoidosis, dermatomyositis, polyarteritis nordosa, scleroderma, giant cell arteritis, cryoglobulinemia), traumatic nerve fiber layer laceration (note: CWS will not resolve), blood diseases (aplastic anemia, dysproteinemia, pernicious anemia [vitamin B12 deficiency]), hyperviscosity syndromes (multiple myeloma, Waldenström macroglobulinemia), hypercoagulability syndromes (factor V Leiden, prothrombin 20210A, hyperhomocysteinemia, protein S/C deficiency, antithrombin III deficiency, dysfibrinogenemia, factor XII deficiency), epiretinal membrane traction, and idiopathic.

3. A thorough history (radiation, chemotherapy, trauma) and review of systems are important to guide the laboratory evaluation. The patient needs a systemic workup for diabetes and hypertension. Initial blood tests include CBC and differential, platelet count, glycosylated hemoglobin, ANA, and HIV antibody test. Depending on the patient's cardiovascular risk factors, a workup looking for cardiac valvular disease, carotid stenosis or deep venous sources of emboli may be done. Infectious workup is based on other systemic symptoms.

4. No treatment is required for the retinopathy. The cotton wool spots resolve spontaneously within 1–2 months.

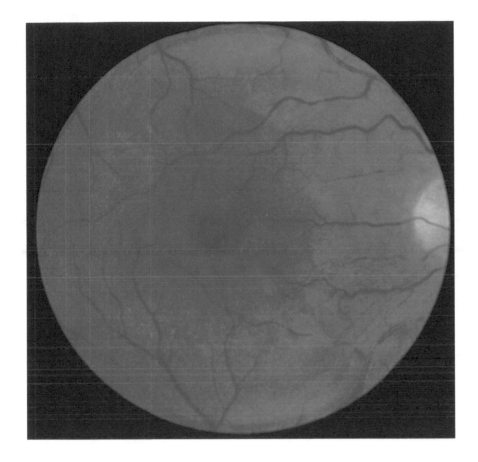

A 67-year-old woman noticed a sudden decrease in vision a few months ago.

1. What is the differential diagnosis?
2. How would you evaluate this patient?
3. How is this entity classified?

1. Macular hole, pseudohole, lamellar hole, cystoid macular edema, solar retinopathy (usually bilateral), epiretinal membrane, and exudative maculopathies including CSC and wet AMD.

2. Perform a dilated fundus examination with evaluation for a Watzke–Allen sign (absolute scotoma over the hole).

   An OCT scan differentiates a macular hole from other entities including lamellar hole, pseudohole, solar retinopathy, cystoid macular edema, CSC, epiretinal membrane, and VMTS. It also illustrates intraretinal abnormalities including cystoid macular edema, intraretinal thickening, and the amount of traction on the edges of the hole. OCT is useful for staging the hole.

   An FA is generally not required to differentiate this entity from others. It would show a window defect corresponding to the hole.

3. *Gass classification* (based on clinical findings):

   Stage 0: VMA or VMT in fellow eye of patient with full-thickness hole.

   Stage 1: premacular or impending hole with foveal detachment, decreased/absent foveal depression, and macular cyst (1A = yellow spot, 100–200 μm in diameter, 1B = yellow ring, 200–300 μm in diameter). There is no PVD, Weiss ring, or vitreofoveal separation. Also known as VMT since no full-thickness defect.

   Stage 2: early, small, full-thickness hole either centrally within the ring or eccentrically at the ring's margin. The OCT shows the partial thickness opening of the hole.

   Stage 3: full-thickness hole (≥300 μm) often with yellow deposits at the level of retinal pigment epithelium (Klein's tags), operculum over the hole within the hyaloid face, cuff of subretinal fluid at hole edges, cystoid macular edema at hole edges, absence of a Weiss ring, and positive Watzke–Allen sign (subjective interruption of slit beam on biomicroscopy).

   Stage 4: stage 3 and PVD.

   International VMT Study Group classification (based on OCT and etiology):

   Primary: full-thickness macular hole (full-thickness defect on OCT)

   Main subclassification: with or without VMT

   Subcategorized by horizontal linear width across FTMH at thinnest point:

   Small: ≤250 μm

   Medium: >250 μm and ≤400 μm

   Large: >400 μm

   Secondary: full-thickness retinal defect from preexisting or concurrent condition including trauma, myopia, macular edema, macular schisis, or surgery.

4. Stage 3 full-thickness macular hole with no VMT.

Additional information: the OCT shows:

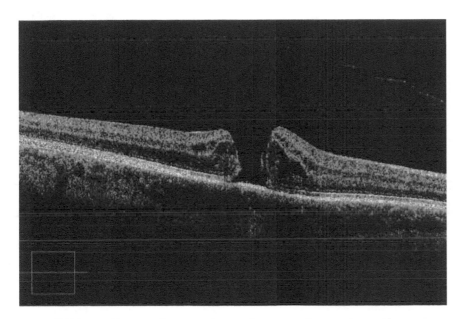

4. What is the diagnosis?

5. What are the risk factors?

6. What is the treatment?

7. What is the prognosis?

5. Cystoid macular edema, VMT on the macula, trauma, postsurgical, postlaser treatment, and postinflammatory disorders.

6. Stage 1 and some stage 2 holes are usually observed for spontaneous release of the hyaloid and hole closure. An intravitreal injection of 0.3 cc of 100% C3F8, an expansile gas (DRCR.net Protocol AG/AH) (pneumatic vitreolysis) or an enzymatic vitreolysis with ocriplasmin (Jetrea) to release the traction can also be used. VMT (stage 1) and small full-thickness holes with traction (stage 2) are candidates for treatment with ocriplasmin especially those < 250 μm. Full thickness macular holes are treated with pars plana vitrectomy with the release of traction from the edges of the hole and placement of a nonexpansile, gas tamponade (usually sulfur hexafluoride) with face-down positioning for several days to 1 week after surgery.

7. The prognosis depends on the duration and size of the hole. It is good for recent onset and smaller diameter holes, as well as patients with good preoperative visual acuity. The prognosis is poor for holes > 1 year duration and > 400 μm wide. Surgery is successful anatomically in 80%–100% of cases depending on duration of the hole and hole width, with 65%–85% of patients gaining three or more lines of visual acuity.

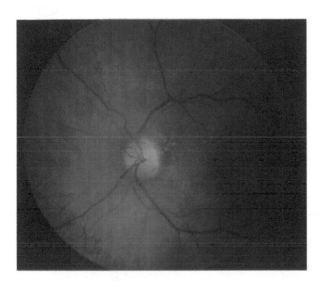

A 53-year-old man complains of photopsias and floaters for 2 days.

1. What finding does he have?
2. What is the diagnosis?
3. What other findings would you look for?
4. If the retinal exam is normal, how would you manage this patient?

Additional information: the patient returns in 1 month with an increase in symptoms and the following peripheral retinal appearance:

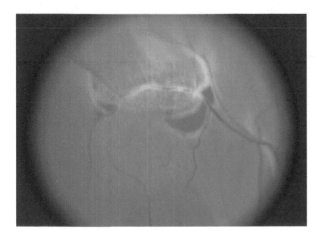

5. What is the diagnosis?
6. What are the risk factors?
7. What is the etiology?
8. What is the treatment?

1. Separation of the posterior hyaloid face from the retina with a Weiss ring.

2. PVD.

3. Retinal break (seen in 10%–15% of acute, symptomatic PVDs) and RRD especially when pigmented anterior vitreous cells are present, and/or vitreous hemorrhage (seen in 7.5% of acute, symptomatic PVDs) from a torn vessel during vitreous separation (70% risk of a retinal tear).

4. Instruct patient in the signs/symptoms of a retinal tear/detachment and repeat a dilated retinal exam in 4–6 weeks.

5. Retinal tear and RRD.

6. Risk factors for retinal tears include age, history of RD in fellow eye (15%), high myopia/axial length (7%), family history, lattice degeneration, trauma, cataract surgery (1% after ICCE; 0.1% after ECCE with intact posterior capsule), diabetes, and Nd:YAG laser posterior capsulotomy.

7. Retinal tears occur when the vitreous detaches posteriorly and reaches a site with firmer attachment. The vitreous remains attached at the posterior margin of the retinal flap creating the horseshoe appearance. With additional traction, retinal tissue may avulse leading to an operculum over a round/oval hole.

8. Horseshoe tears and symptomatic retinal holes should be treated with laser photocoagulation or cryopexy to prevent RD. Asymptomatic retinal holes can be observed. In this case, the patient has developed a RRD that requires surgical repair. If the tears are superior and localized to 1 clock hour, the patient is a candidate for pneumatic retinopexy. If not, a scleral buckle or primary pars plana vitrectomy should be performed.

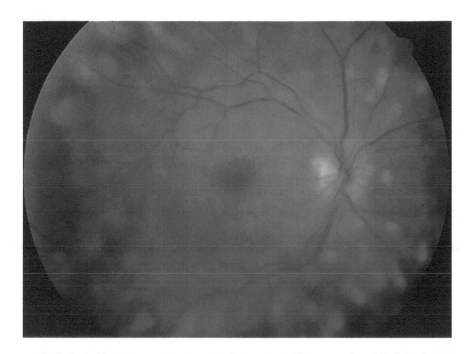

A 57-year-old woman complains of blurred vision, nyctalopia, and peripheral photopsias in both eyes for 3 days.

1. What does the fundus photo show?
2. What is the differential diagnosis?
3. What ancillary studies would you obtain to make the diagnosis?

Additional information: laboratory testing reveals patient is positive for HLA-A29.

4. What is the diagnosis?
5. What other exam findings would you look for?
6. What is the epidemiology of this disease?
7. How would you treat this patient?
8. What is the prognosis?

1. Multiple, small, discrete, ovoid, creamy yellow-white spots at the level of the choroid and RPE scattered like a birdshot blast from a shotgun in the midperiphery radiating from the optic nerve. Notably, the lesions are not pigmented.

2. The differential diagnosis includes inflammatory disorders such as birdshot chorioretinopathy, other white dot syndromes (MEWDS, APMPPE), pars planitis, punctate inner choroidopathy, and sarcoidosis; infectious etiologies such as tuberculosis, syphilis, DUSN, and toxoplasmosis; masquerade processes such as ocular lymphoma, metastatic disease, and choroidal lymphoproliferative diseases.

3. Laboratory testing for HLA typing would be most useful.

   FA is useful to characterize the lesions. Birdshot lesions show mild hyperfluorescence early (active lesions may hypofluoresce early) and late staining. Late views show profuse vascular incompetence with leakage, petalloid CME, and secondary retinal staining. The phenomena of "quenching," where dye seems to disappear rapidly from the retinal circulation, can also be seen in these patients. ICG shows characteristic hypofluorescent dark dots in the intermediate phase of the angiogram and late-diffuse choroidal hyperfluorescence.

4. Birdshot chorioretinopathy, also known as vitiliginous chorioretinitis, is associated with HLA-A29 (90%–98%), although 7% of the general population is positive for HLA-A29.

5. Other signs of birdshot include mild vitritis, mild anterior chamber cells and flare (in 25% of cases), CME, retinal vasculitis, and variable amount of disc edema. Late findings include optic atrophy and epiretinal membranes. Macular CNV is rare.

6. Birdshot chorioretinopathy is a rare uveitis that occurs mainly in 50- to 60-year-old females (70%) and almost exclusively in Caucasians of northern European descent.

7. Treatment is reserved for patients with decreased visual acuity, significant inflammation, or complications including CME.

   Despite historically poor responses to steroids, initial improvement can be seen with oral steroids. Intravitreal or subTenon steroid injection is performed in patients with severe inflammation or CME. Early introduction of steroid-sparing agents, immunomodulatory agents including cyclosporine, azathioprine, mycophenolate mofetil, adalimumab, daclizumab, methotrexate, or IV polyclonal immunoglobulin can also be considered.

8. Birdshot is a chronic, slowly progressive, recurrent disease with variable visual prognosis. Most patients lose vision from chronic CME. Rarely, it is a self-limited disease.

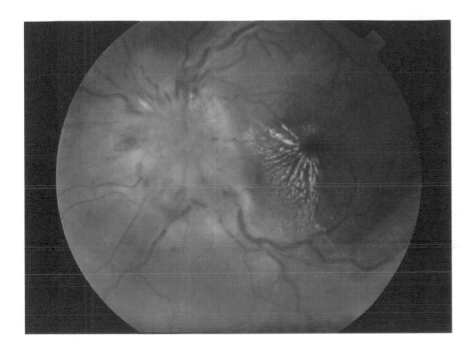

A 28-year-old woman reports sudden vision loss in her left eye after having flu-like symptoms the week before.

1. What findings are shown?
2. What is the differential diagnosis?
3. How would you work up this patient?

Additional information: laboratory testing is positive for B. henselae.

4. What is the diagnosis?
5. How would you treat this patient?
6. What is the prognosis?

1. Marked optic disc edema with disc hemorrhage and lipid exudation in a star shape.

2. The patient has a macular star exudate. Infectious etiologies to consider and rule out include *B. henselae*, syphillis, Lyme disease, tuberculosis, tularemia, toxoplasmosis, viral retinitis (HSV, VZV, EBV), DUSN, and toxocariasis. Noninfectious etiologies to consider include hypertensive retinopathy, diabetic retinopathy, AION, retinal vein occlusion, acute macular neuroretinopathy, sarcoidosis, and papilledema.

3. Check blood pressure. Laboratory testing for VDRL or RPR, FTA-ABS or MHA-TP, PPD, and IFA for *B. henselae*.

4. Neuroretinitis, also known as Leber idiopathic stellate neuroretinitis, is due to a pleomorphic, Gram-negative bacillus called *B. henselae* (formerly known as *Rochalimaea*), which is associated with cat-scratch disease.

5. There are no definitive treatment guidelines given the self-limited nature of the disease and good prognosis. The use of systemic antibiotics (doxycycline, rifampin, tetracycline, ciprofloxacin, trimethoprim [Bactrim]) and steroids is controversial. The typical regimen for an immunocompetent patient is doxycycline for 2–4 weeks. For severe infections, IV doxycycline can be given along with rifampin.

6. Good with 67% regaining ≥ 20/20 vision, and 97% regaining > 20/40 vision. The disc edema resolves over 8–12 weeks, whereas the macular star takes longer, resolving over 6–12 months. Optic atrophy and retinal pigment epithelial changes may develop late.

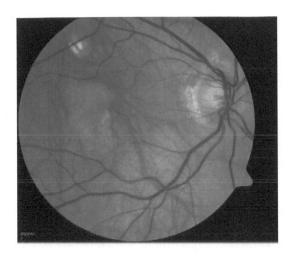

A 45-year-old man complains of blurred vision with metamorphopsia.

1. What does the photo depict?
2. What is the differential diagnosis?
3. What ancillary tests would you order?
4. What is the diagnosis?
5. What are the risk factors for this disease?
6. What other clinical findings are common?

Additional information: the FA shows:

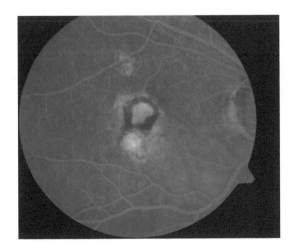

7. How would you treat this patient?
8. What is the prognosis?

1. Small, round, yellow-brown, punched-out chorioretinal lesions (histo-spots) in the midperiphery and posterior pole, and juxtapapillary atrophic changes. In the macula there is a pigmented chorioretinal scar with CNV. The media is notably clear, indicating no vitreous haze.

2. In a patient of this age, CNV is usually due to POHS, pathologic myopia, or an inflammatory disorder such as multifocal choroiditis or punctate inner chorioretinopathy.

3. To verify that a CNV is present, FA is most useful. OCT or OCTA would also show the CNV. Laboratory testing is largely unnecessary, although histoplasmin antigen skin testing can be performed. It is important to note that 60% of the adult population of the Ohio and Mississippi River Valleys has a positive reaction to histoplasmin skin testing.

4. POHS, caused by previous infection by the dimorphic fungus *Histoplasma capsulatum*, with secondary CNV.

5. Endemic in the Ohio and Mississippi river valleys, the fungus is present on the feathers of chickens, pigeons, and blackbirds, in addition to infected bat droppings. Humans inhale fungus, which then disseminates into the bloodstream. POHS is rare in African Americans. It is associated with HLA-B7.

6. Over 60% of cases are bilateral. Most patients are asymptomatic unless they develop CNV. The four characteristic findings of POHS are: punched-out chorioretinal lesions (histo-spots), peripapillary atrophic pigmentary changes, lack of vitritis, and CNV.

7. *Laser:* extra- and juxtafoveal CNV can be treated with focal laser photocoagulation. Subfoveal CNV should not be treated with laser (14% regress spontaneously).
   Photodynamic therapy (PDT): subfoveal CNV can be treated with ocular PDT with verteporfin (Visudyne).
   Anti-vascular endothelial growth factor (anti-VEGF): although there are no randomized studies and no FDA-approved therapies for POHS, anti-VEGF agents (ranibizumab, bevacizumab, aflibercept, brolucizumab, pegaptanib) are the first-line treatment of POHS-related CNV with good success off-label.
   Surgery: removal of CNV with subretinal surgery was evaluated in Subretinal Surgery Trials (Group H); however, surgery was not found to be beneficial in patients with vision better than 20/100. Patients with vision worse than 20/100 had a better chance of improving vision over 2 years of follow-up. There was a high rate of CNV recurrence, cataract formation, and retinal detachment. Surgery has largely been supplanted by anti-VEGF injections.

8. Better visual prognosis than CNV due to age-related macular degeneration with a 30% recurrence rate. Patients are at risk for CNV in the fellow eye (risk is < 2% per year).

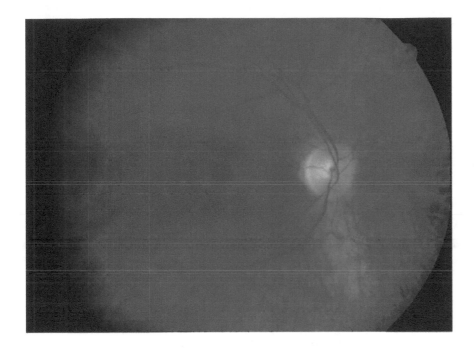

A 48-year-old woman has bilateral chronic vision loss.

1. What finding is present?
2. What is the differential diagnosis?
3. What tests would you obtain?
4. What other history would be helpful?

Additional information: the patient is being treated for SLE for 15 years.

5. What is the most likely diagnosis?
6. What are the risk factors for this problem?
7. How would you follow this patient?
8. How would you treat this patient?
9. What is the prognosis?

1. Retinal pigment epithelium depigmentation in a "bull's eye" configuration.

2. The differential diagnosis of a "bull's eye" maculopathy includes cone and cone–rod dystrophy, AMD, Stargardt disease/fundus flavimaculatus, central areolar choroidal dystrophy, benign concentric annular dystrophy, chloroquine/hydroxychloroquine retinal toxicity, chronic macular hole, olivopontocerebellar atrophy, and ceroid lipofuscinosis.

3. FA would demonstrate the "bull's eye" pattern of hypofluorescence with a ring of hyperfluorescence that is often visible before the fundus lesion. It would rule out the "dark choroid" seen in Stargardt disease. Fundus autofluorescence would also demonstrate the bull's eye pattern. Humphrey visual field central 10 degrees (10–2) white-on-white pattern may demonstrate visual field defects. Multifocal ERG would show central depression. OCT shows thinning of the retina in the area of the bull's eye with absent inner/outer segment junction in a ring pattern (called flying saucer sign), which is very characteristic and obviates the need for FA in many patients. En-face OCT views are also helpful to see the bull's eye pattern.

4. It is important to ask the patient specifically about SLE, rheumatoid arthritis, short-term pulse treatment for graft-versus-host disease and amebiasis, the use of toxic medications such as quinolones, and a history of any relatives with a similar eye problem to rule out a hereditary maculopathy.

5. Hydroxychloroquine retinal toxicity. Quinolones, first used as an antimalarial agent in World War II, are now used to treat SLE, rheumatoid arthritis, short-term pulse treatment for graft-versus-host disease, and amebiasis.

6. The major risk factors for retinal toxicity are daily dosage (most important; >5.0 mg/kg real weight for hydroxychloroquine, >2.3 mg/kg real weight for chloroquine), duration of use (>5 years with no other risk factors), renal disease, and concomitant tamoxifen use (5 × increased risk). Other risk factors include liver disease, older age, and retinal/macular disease. The prevalence of toxicity is 7.5% among long-term users. The risk of developing hydroxychloroquine toxicity at recommended doses (<5.0 mg/kg/day) is < 1% up to 5 years, <2% up to 10 years, and ~20% after 20 years.

7. The 2016 revised American Academy of Ophthalmology recommendations on screening are as follows: a baseline ophthalmic exam within a year of starting the medication, and visual field and spectral domain OCT if there is a maculopathy. Annual screenings beginning after 5 years of medication use or sooner if patient has major risk factors. High-risk patients should be checked more frequently.

   Recommended screening tests: primary tests are automated visual fields (10-2 for non-Asians, paracentral scotoma; 24-2 or 30-2 for Asians, scotoma extends beyond macula) and/or spectral domain OCT (ring of outer retinal thinning; flying saucer sign), and other objective tests are mfERG (enlarged a-wave, depressed b-wave) and FAF (reduced).

   Not recommended for screening are fundus examination, time domain OCT, FA, full-field ERG, Amsler grid, color testing, and EOG.

8. There is no treatment for hydroxychloroquine toxicity. Decrease or discontinue the medication to prevent central vision loss.

9. Retinopathy is not reversible and can even progress after the drug is discontinued.

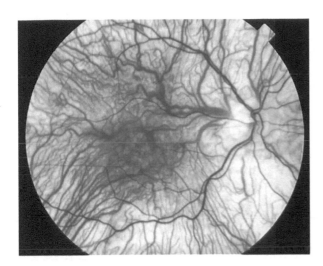

A 19-year-old college student sees you for a new glasses prescription.

1. What does the photo reveal?
2. What is the differential diagnosis?
3. What other eye findings would you look for?

Additional information: slit-lamp examination with retroillumination shows:

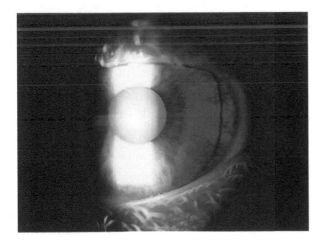

4. What is the diagnosis?
5. Describe the forms of this disease.
6. What are the risk factors for this disease?
7. How would you treat this patient?
8. What is the prognosis?

1. Generalized fundus hypopigmentation with the deep choroidal vasculature visible. There is foveal hypoplasia with no luteal pigment or foveal light reflex present.

2. Blond fundus (variant of normal) or ocular albinism.

3. Decreased vision, photophobia, high myopia, nystagmus, strabismus, pale irides with diffuse transillumination.

4. Ocular albinism.

5. Albinism is a congenital disorder of melanogenesis in which the synthesis of melanin is reduced or absent. Mutations in at least 13 genes can give rise to various forms of albinism depending on which structures are involved:

    Ocular albinism: this is a disorder, limited to the eye, with a decreased number of melanosomes (although each melanosome is fully pigmented).

    Oculocutaneous albinism: this is a systemic problem with decreased melanin in all melanosomes. These patients lack pigmentation of the hair, skin, and eyes. This form can further be categorized into tyrosinase positive (some pigmentation, which increases with age) and tyrosinase negative (no pigmentation). Two lethal variants of oculocutaneous albinism are:

    > **Chediak–Higashi**: patients have reticuloendothelial incompetence with neutropenia, anemia, thrombocytopenia, recurrent infections, leukemia, and lymphoma.

    > **Hermansky–Pudlak**: patients have clotting disorders and bleeding tendencies secondary to platelet abnormalities.

    All of the above forms of albinism can be further classified clinically based on the degree of ocular involvement:

    > True albinism: patients have low visual acuity 20/100 to 20/400) and nystagmus due to hypoplasia of the fovea.

    > Albinoidism: patients have normal or only slightly diminished visual acuity without nystagmus.

6. This is a heritable disease. Certain ethnic populations have a higher incidence. In particular, Africans and African Americans have a higher incidence than Caucasians, but often have incomplete forms of albinism.

7. There is no effective treatment. Refraction, tinted glasses, and low-vision aids are helpful for older patients. Medical and hematology consultation is advisable to rule out potentially lethal variants. All forms of albinism are heritable, necessitating genetic counseling.

8. The prognosis is variable depending on the form of albinism. This disease is not degenerative, however, and visual acuity can even improve over the first two decades of life.

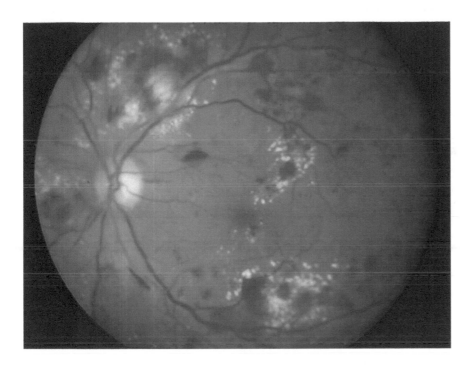

A 36-year-old man presents with decreased vision in his left eye.

1. What are the retinal findings?

2. What is the most likely diagnosis and what tests can be performed to confirm it?

3. What is the differential diagnosis?

4. What additional ophthalmic tests would be helpful?

5. What level of retinopathy does this patient exhibit?

1. Numerous intraretinal hemorrhages, microaneurysms, cotton-wool spots, and lipid exudates scattered throughout the posterior pole. No retinal or optic nerve neovascularization, preretinal hemorrhage, or vitreous hemorrhage is seen.

2. Diabetic retinopathy. Check serum hemoglobin A1c, fasting blood sugar, and blood pressure.

3. Hypertensive retinopathy, retinopathies associated with blood disorders, radiation retinopathy, retinal vein occlusion, ocular ischemic syndrome, parafoveal telangiectasia, and Eales disease.

4. FA would be useful to evaluate macular ischemia and to rule out neovascularization. OCT scan would be useful to evaluate for the presence of posterior hyaloidal traction, epiretinal proliferation, and the nature of the macular edema (diffuse versus focal). OCTA can show retinal ischemia and microaneurysms.

5. Diabetic retinopathy can be classified based on the clinical features. This patient has very severe nonproliferative diabetic retinopathy (NPDR) defined by the "4-2-1 rule": (4) intraretinal hemorrhages and/or microaneurysms in all four quadrants; or (2) venous beading in at least 2 quadrants; or (1) IRMA in at least one quadrant. Very severe NPDR exists if there is more than one of these features, as in this case.

6. How would you manage this patient?

7. This patient has proliferative diabetic retinopathy in his fellow eye. How would you treat it?

6. *Medical*: the DCCT and UKPDS concluded that tight blood sugar and blood pressure control slowed the progression of retinopathy, development of macular edema, need for treatment, and other microvascular complications.

   Anti-VEGF: for macular edema involving the fovea (center-involving), ranibizumab (Lucentis; DCR. net Protocol I, DRCR.net Protocol T, DRCR net Protocol S, RISE, RIDE, RESTORE, and RESOLVE studies), aflibercept (Eylea; DRCR.net Protocol T, DRCR.net Protocol W, VIVID, VISTA studies, PANORAMA), bevacizumab (Avastin; DRCR.net Protocol T), brolucizumab (Beovu; KITE and KESTREL studies), and faricimab (Vabysmo; YOSEMITE and RHINE studies) have been shown to be very effective therapies. This patient would be an ideal candidate for intravitreal anti-VEGF therapy. Protocol T suggests that if the vision was < 20/50, then aflibercept may be the best choice, but if the vision was better, then any of the three anti-VEGF agents would work. In year 2 of Protocol T, there was no difference between aflibercept and ranibizumab, but bevacizumab was not as effective. KITE/KESTREL showed that brolucizumab was noninferior to every 8-week aflibercept but at a 8- to 12-week dosing intervals, while faricimab in YOSEMITE and RHINE showed similar efficacy to every 8-week aflibercept but at 12- to 16-week dosing intervals.

   Laser: the EDTRS concluded that focal/grid laser photocoagulation decreased moderate visual loss by 50% in patients with CSME defined as: (1) retinal thickening within 500 μm of the macular center *or* (2) hard exudates within 500 μm of the macular center with adjacent thickening *or* (3) zone of retinal thickening 1 disc area in size any portion of which is within 1 disc diameter of the macular center. CSME is based only on clinical examination and not visual acuity (treat even with 20/20 vision) or other imaging studies. Laser treatment is second line to anti-VEGF therapy.

   Steroids: considered third-line therapy behind laser and anti-VEGF therapy, intraocular steroids have been shown to be effective especially in patients who are already pseudophakic. Although the DRCR.net Protocol B did not find steroids better than laser in the overall study population, DRCR.net Protocol I did show a benefit in pseudophakic patients. Similarly, the sustained-release, fluocinolone acetonide steroid implant (Iluvien) has been shown to be effective over a 3-year follow-up period in patients who had previous laser therapy and persistent edema (FAME Study). Finally, the dexamthesone implant (Ozuredex) has been found to be effective (MEAD Study). With all steroids, careful monitoring of cataract formation and IOP is important.

   Surgery: if a patient exhibits posterior hyaloidal traction, then pars plana vitrectomy with membrane peel should be considered. This patient did not exhibit any traction.

7. The first question would be to decide if the patient had high-risk characteristics or not.

   High-risk characteristics of PDR are defined as: neovascularization of the disc (NVD) > standard photo 10A used in DRS (1/3 to 1/4 disc area) *or* any NVD and VH or preretinal hemorrhage *or* neovascularization elsewhere (NVE) > standard photo 7 (1/2 disc area) and VH or preretinal hemorrhage.

   The DRS concluded that, in the presence of high-risk characteristics, immediate PRP should be instituted. However, the DRCR.net Protocol S showed that ranibizumab was noninferior to PRP in patients with PDR. Patients treated with ranibizumab had better visual field outcomes at 2 years but not at 5 years, less center-involved DME, and lower rates of retinal detachment. In Protocol AB, aflibercept injections gave similar outcomes to vitrectomy with endolaser for patients with vitreous hemorrhage and PDR. Thus, treatment with anti-VEGF injection in patients with moderate to severe NPDR improves diabetic retinopathy severity and reduces the risk of progression to vision-threatening complications and DME. It is also an option in PDR.

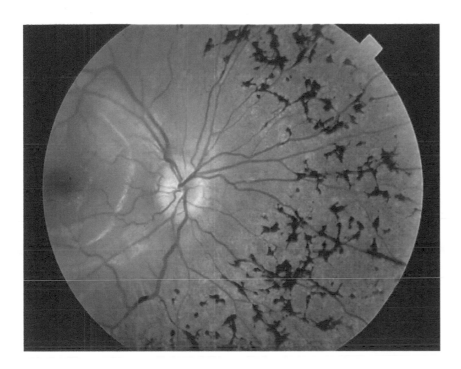

A 26-year-old man says he has noted trouble with night driving.

1. What does the picture show?
2. What is the differential diagnosis?

Additional examination: ERG shows markedly reduced/absent a-wave and b-wave amplitudes and implicit times.

3. What is the diagnosis?
4. What other eye findings are associated with this disease?

1. Dark pigmentary clumps in the midperiphery and perivenous areas (bone spicules), attenuated retinal vessels, and waxy optic disc pallor.

2. Bone spicules and disc pallor are found in RP, congenital rubella syndrome, syphilis, thioridazine/chloroquine drug toxicity, carcinoma-associated retinopathy, congenital stationary night blindness, vitamin A deficiency, trauma, and diffuse unilateral subacute neuroretinitis.

3. RP.

4. Posterior subcapsular cataracts, high myopia, astigmatism, keratoconus, constricted visual fields, dyschromatopsia, and mild hearing loss (30%, excluding patients with Usher syndrome). Fifty percent of female carriers with the X-linked form have a golden reflex in the posterior pole.

5. Describe the various forms of this disease and their classification.

5. There are more than 29 loci associated with various phenotypes of RP, with more being discovered daily.
    Atypical forms:

    RP inversus: the macula and posterior pole are primarily affected, so this form is confused with hereditary macular disorders. Central and color vision are reduced earlier than normal and pericentral ring/central scotomas occur.

    RP sine pigmento: this is a descriptive term for patients with symptoms of RP, but who fail to show pigmentary fundus changes. It is seen in up to 20% of cases and is associated with more pronounced cone dysfunction.

    Retinitis punctata albescens (AR): multiple, punctate white (50–100 µm) spots at the level of the RPE are scattered in the midperiphery with attenuated vessels and bone spicules. This is a slowly progressive disease, which differentiates it from fundus albipunctatus.

    Sector RP: this form has pigmentary changes limited to one retinal area that generally does not enlarge, usually in the inferonasal quadrants, and therefore the ERG responses are relatively good.

    Forms associated with systemic abnormalities:

    Abetalipoproteinemia (Bassen–Kornzweig syndrome; AR): this form has minimal pigmentary changes early and is associated with ataxia, steatorrhea, erythrocyte acanthocytosis, growth retardation, neuropathy, and lack of serum beta-lipoprotein causing intestinal malabsorption of fat-soluble vitamins (A, D, E, K), triglycerides, and cholesterol.

    Alstrom disease (AR): this form has early profound visual loss and is associated with cataracts, deafness, obesity, renal failure, acanthosis nigricans, baldness, and hypogenitalism.

    Cockayne syndrome: this form is associated with band keratopathy, cataracts, dwarfism, deafness, intracranial calcifications, and psychosis.

    Kearns–Sayre syndrome (AR): this form is associated with chronic, progressive external ophthalmoplegia, ptosis, cardiac conduction defects (arrhythmias, heart block, cardiomyopathy), and other abnormalities. "Ragged red" fibers are seen histologically on muscle biopsy.

    Laurence–Moon/Bardet–Biedl syndrome (AR): Bardet–Biedl (polydactyly in 75% and syndactyly in 14%) and Laurence–Moon (spastic paraplegia, no polydactyly/syndactyly). Both forms have minimal pigmentary changes early and are characterized by short stature, congenital obesity, hypogenitalism (50%), partial deafness (5%), renal abnormalities, and mental retardation (85%).

    Neuronal ceroid lipofuscinosis (Batten disease) (AR): this form can have infantile (Hagberg–Santavuori syndrome), juvenile, or adult onset and is associated with seizures, dementia, ataxia, and mental retardation. Conjunctival biopsy shows granular inclusions with autofluorescent lipopigments that also accumulate in neurons causing the retinal and CNS degeneration.

    Refsum disease (AR): this form has minimal pigmentary changes early and is associated with ichthyosis, electrocardiogram abnormalities, anosmia, deafness, progressive peripheral neuropathy, cerebellar ataxia, hypotonia, hepatomegaly, mental retardation, and elevated cerebrospinal fluid protein. It is caused by a defect in fatty acid metabolism due to phytanic acid oxidase deficiency. This results in elevated plasma phytanic acid, pipecolic acid, and very long-chain fatty acid levels.

    Usher syndrome (AR): this form is associated with congenital, neurosensory hearing loss. It is the most common syndrome associated with RP (5%), and there are 4 types: type I (total deafness with no vestibular function), type II (partial deafness with normal vestibular function, most common type (67%), better vision), type III (Hallgren syndrome = deafness, vestibular ataxia, psychosis), and type IV (deafness and mental retardation).

6. How would you treat this patient?

7. What is the prognosis?

6. For most forms including this patient there is no effective treatment, but some patients respond to oral vitamin A therapy (slows reduction of ERG amplitudes) and avoidance of vitamin E. When patients are placed on this therapy, liver function tests and serum retinol levels should be checked annually. In addition, treatment should include obtaining the best visual potential for the patient including correcting any refractive error, prescribing dark glasses, and low vision consultation for visual aids.

7. The prognosis is usually poor. Most patients are legally blind by the 4th decade of life.

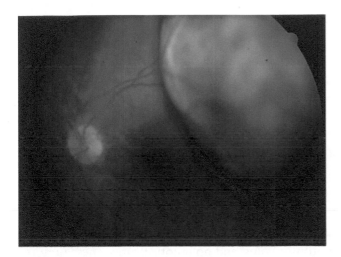

A 70-year-old man presents with blurred vision in his left eye. He notes having intermittent photopsias over the past 3 months in that eye but became concerned when he developed a visual field defect.

1. What does the photo reveal?
2. What etiology do you suspect?
3. What other tests would you order?

Additional information: a fine-needle biopsy is obtained.

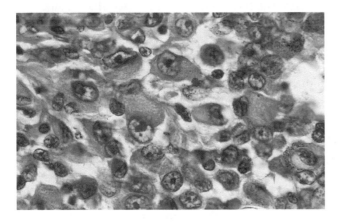

4. What does the pathology show?
5. What is the recommended treatment?
6. How would you follow this patient after treatment?
7. What is the prognosis?
8. What are the complications of radiation therapy?

1. A brown, domed-shaped mass with overlying exudative retinal detachment.

2. Choroidal malignant melanoma.

3. The most important test is ultrasound to differentiate between a tumor and other diseases in the differential diagnosis. B-scan would show the tumor and the shape of the tumor (eg, mushroom, dome, or biconvex shape). A-scan in a choroidal malignant melanoma would show low to medium internal reflectivity with reduction in amplitude from front to back, and high-amplitude spikes consistent with break in Bruch membrane. Careful examination must be performed to evaluate for extrascleral extension. FA would show "double" circulation within the tumor from filling of both the retinal and choroidal vasculature. The lesion itself would be hypofluorescent early with pinpoint leakage late. Although not required, neuroimaging can be performed (a melanoma is bright on T1 and dark on T2 MRI imaging).

4. This specimen demonstrates epithelioid cells. Histopathology is based on the *Callender classification:*

    Spindle A cells: slender with cigar-shaped nucleus and finely dispersed chromatin. They have a low nuclear-to-cytoplasmic ratio, absent or inconspicuous nucleolus, and no mitotic figures. These tumors carry the best prognosis (5-year survival rate = 95%).

    Spindle B cells: oval with larger nucleus containing mitotic figures and coarser chromatin and prominent nucleolus.

    Epithelioid cells: polyhedral with abundant cytoplasm and a large, round-to-oval nucleus with peripheral margination of chromatin and prominent eosinophilic or purple nucleolus. The cells are poorly cohesive with distinct borders. Epithelioid cells are the most malignant and carry the worst prognosis (5-year survival < 30%).

5. This patient should be treated with enucleation.

    Treatment is based on the size of the tumor defined in the Collaborative Ocular Melanoma Study (COMS):

    Small tumors (apical height = 1.5–2.4 mm and basal diameter = 5–16 mm): there is no clear treatment choice, so these tumors can be observed closely if they are very small. Risk factors for growth of small melanomas are based on the following findings: thickness > 2 mm, subretinal fluid, symptoms, orange pigment, margin < 3 mm from optic disc, ultrasound hollow, halo absent, drusen absent (0 factors risk = 4%, each risk increases relative risk approximately 3 ×).

    Medium tumors (apical height = 2.5–10 mm and basal diameter ≤ 16 mm): since survival rates were similar between enucleation and iodine-125 plaque brachytherapy, the treatment of choice is radiation with either a high-energy radiation source (cobalt-60, iridium-192), low-energy radiation source (iodine-125, palladium-106, ruthenium-106), or charged particle radiation (proton beam).

    Large tumors (apical height > 10 mm and basal diameter > 16 mm; without metastasis. Updated definition is apical height > 2 mm and basal diameter > 16 mm, or apical height > 10 mm regardless of basal diameter, or apical height > 8 mm and < 2 mm from optic disc): since preenucleation radiation did not change the survival rate in patients with large choroidal melanomas with or without metastases over enucleation alone, the treatment of choice is enucleation.

6. Patients need to be observed closely for metastasis. The most common sites of metastasis are the liver, lung, bone, skin, and CNS; therefore, annual liver function tests and chest imaging should be performed.

7. Approximately 50% of patients with large tumors have metastasis within 5 years with a mean survival after metastasis of 9 months.

8. The main complications are radiation retinopathy, cataracts (posterior subcapsular in 42% within 3 years of proton beam therapy), and dry eye. There is a high risk of substantial visual loss from iodine-125 brachytherapy (up to 49%) and patients must understand that the therapy is to treat the tumor and not vision.

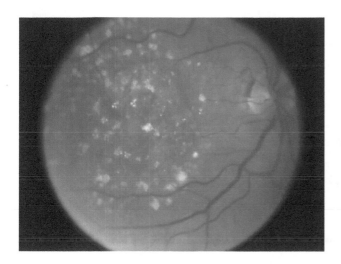 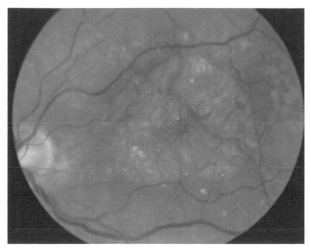

A 68-year-old man reports a gradual decline in vision for years. His visual acuity is 20/60 OD and 20/200 OS. He is interested in cataract surgery to correct his vision.

1. What retinal findings are present and what is the diagnosis?

2. What risk factors are associated with this disease?

3. What tests would be helpful?

1. Dry AMD with drusen and RPE changes in the macula OD and geographic atrophy OS.

2. Risk factors include age (>75 years), positive family history, smoking, hyperopia, light iris color, hypertension, hypercholesterolemia, cardiovascular disease, and female gender.

3. Pinhole vision, near vision, refraction, Amsler grid testing, and potential acuity meter can help assess the visual potential prior to cataract surgery. OCT should be obtained to rule out exudative changes (ie, pigment epithelium detachment, subretinal fluid). If wet AMD is detected, then FA or OCTA is useful to verify the presence of a choroidal neovascular membrane. ICG angiography can also be considered.

4. The OCT reveals drusen without exudate confirming the diagnosis of dry AMD. Fundus photos and OCT are used to document and follow progression. Treatment consists of oral supplements (AREDS or

Additional information: the OCT shows:

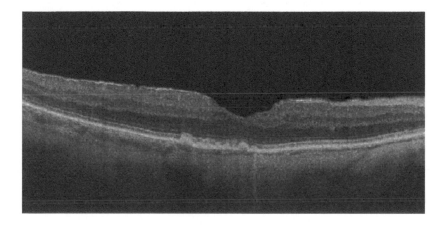

4. How would you treat this patient?
5. Discuss the AREDS findings.
6. What is the prognosis?

AREDS2 formulation depending on smoking status) and vision self-monitoring with an Amsler grid. The patient should return for evaluation if he notices any change in the appearance of the Amsler grid. There is currently no therapy for geographic atrophy but low-vision aids may be helpful. There are numerous drugs in phase 3 clinical testing to reduce the risk of GA progression mainly through complement cascade modulation.

5. The AREDS reported that supplements with high-dose antioxidants and zinc (vitamin C 500 mg; vitamin E 400 IU; and beta carotene 15 mg, zinc 80 mg, and copper 2 mg) are helpful in reducing vision loss and the progression of disease in patients with category 3 and 4 AMD. The *AREDS classification* is:

   Category 1: fewer than five small (<63 μm) drusen.

   Category 2 (mild AMD): multiple small drusen or single or nonextensive intermediate (63–124 μm) drusen, or pigment abnormalities.

   Category 3 (intermediate AMD): extensive intermediate-sized drusen, or one or more large (>125 μm) drusen, or noncentral geographic atrophy.

   Category 4 (advanced AMD): vision loss (<20/32) due to AMD in one eye (due to either central/subfoveal geographic atrophy or exudative AMD).

   The AREDS2, which evaluated lutein, zeaxanthin, and omega-3 fatty acids in addition to the original AREDS formulation, found that current smokers should avoid high-dose beta carotene (increased risk of lung cancer), adding lutein and zeaxanthin is beneficial (~20% reduction in disease progression beyond original AREDS in patients who had the lowest dietary intake of lutein and zeaxanthin), and there was no additional benefit from omega-3 fatty acids. As a result, the AREDS formula was adjusted by removing beta carotene and adding lutein and zeaxanthin.

6. The rate of progression to advanced AMD over 5 years was 1.3% in eyes with many small or few medium drusen (if both eyes have many intermediate drusen, but no large drusen, then patient score = 1 in scale below), and 18% in eyes with many medium or any large drusen (as in this patient).

   Another method to calculate risk is the AREDS Clinical Severity Scale that is based on giving one point for the presence of ≥ 1 large drusen and/or pigment changes (either hyper, hypo, or noncentral GA) per eye, or 2 points for advanced AMD in one eye, then total the points for the two eyes to obtain a point score that shows the risk of developing advanced AMD in 5 years:

   0 points = 0.5%

   1 point = 3%

   2 points = 12%

   3 points = 25%

   4 points = 50%

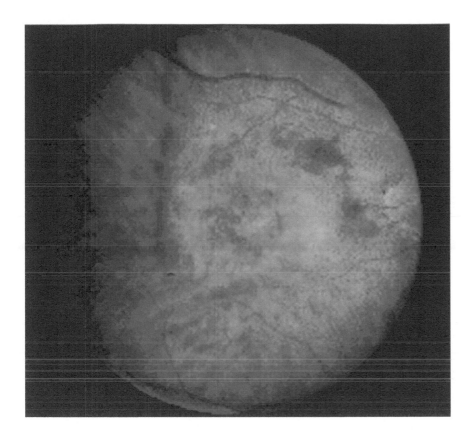

An 85 year old woman presents with new distortion of vision in her right eye.

1. What does the photo show?
2. What is the differential diagnosis?
3. What tests would you perform?

1. Subretinal fluid and hemorrhage.

2. In a patient this age, the differential diagnosis includes exudative AMD, atypical CSC, adult vitelliform lesion, and other causes of CNV including POHS, inflammatory, pathologic myopia, and idiopathic.

3. The key test is FA to verify the presence of a choroidal neovascular membrane and rule out other causes of fluid and hemorrhage. ICG angiography would be useful to evaluate for CSC and PCV. Finally, OCT would verify the presence of fluid, CNV, and rule out other causes such as a thickened choroid with CSC, or a vitelliform lesion. OCTA would also show CNV and help differentitate from other diseases. In general, OCT with OCTA can be used instead of FA and ICG in most cases.

4. Exudative AMD.

5. Since the CNV is subfoveal, the patient is not a candidate for laser photocoagulation:

Additional information: the FA shows:

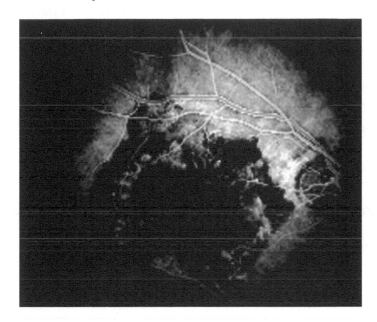

4. What is the most likely diagnosis?

5. What treatment would you recommend?

6. How would you follow this patient?

Anti-VEGF: for CNV involving the fovea, ranibizumab (Lucentis; MARINA, ANCHOR, CATT, IVAN, MANTA, GEFAL studies), bevacizumab (Avastin; CATT, IVAN, MANTA, GEFAL studies), aflibercept (Eylea; VIEW studies), brolucizumab (Beovu; HAWK, HARRIER studies), faricimab (Vabysmo; TENAYA/LUCERNE studies), and the ranibizumab port delivery system (PDS, ARCHWAY study) have been shown to be equally effective therapies but differ in dosing frequency. The PDS is a surgically implanted device with in-office refills every 6 months. Pegaptanib (Macugen) does not have similar visual results as the other anti-VEGF agents and is not first-line therapy. This patient would be a candidate for anti-VEGF therapy.

Ocular PDT with verteporfin (Visudyne): can be used alone (TAP, VIP studies) or in combination with anti-VEGF agents (DENALI, MT BLANC studies) with results of combination therapy similar to anti-VEGF alone. In general, PDT is a second-line therapy unless patient has PCV, where it may offer benefits compared with anti-VEGF alone.

6. The CATT study reported that as-needed therapy gives similar results to monthly therapy but required monthly monitoring. Thus, monthly monitoring with clinical examination and OCT evaluation should be performed to evaluate for evidence of CNV activity. Retreatment should be performed when there is evidence of disease activity. Many physicians also use a treat-and-extend paradigm of treatment (TREX, ALTAIR, ARIES studies).

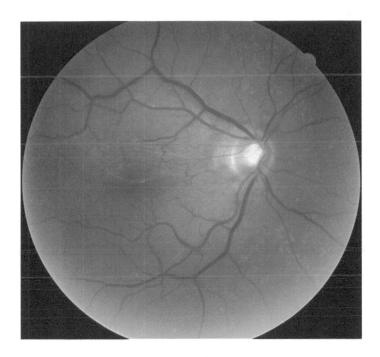

A 63-year-old woman is frustrated because of increasing difficulty reading the newspaper over the past 6 months.

1. What retinal findings are shown?
2. What symptoms may occur?
3. How would you evaluate this patient?

1. There is a thin, translucent membrane with dragged/tortuous vessels and retinal striae especially evident in the superior macula.

2. Metamorphopsia, macropsia, and decreased vision.

3. Visual acuity and Amsler grid testing is useful for monitoring the effect on visual function.

   OCT scan demonstrates the amount of traction produced and differentiates this from other entities including lamellar hole, pseudohole, macular hole, and VMTS. It also illustrates intraretinal abnormalities including cystoid macular edema, intraretinal thickening, and subretinal fluid.

   FA shows the degree of retinal vascular tortuosity, retinal vascular leakage, and macular edema. The presence of macular edema may indicate a worse visual prognosis.

Additional information: her OCT shows:

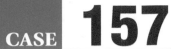

Exam Date:	6/11/2008
Exam Time:	1:04 PM
Technician:	Operator, Cirrus
Signal Strength:	6/10

C.ZMI

Macular Thickness:Macular Cube 200x200   OD ● | ○ OS

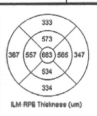

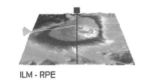

ILM-RPE Thickness (um)

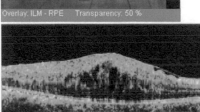

Overlay: ILM - RPE   Transparency: 50 %

ILM - RPE

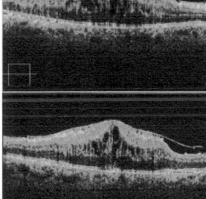

ILM

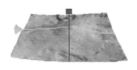

RPE

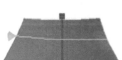

	Central Subfield Thickness um	Volume mm3	Average Thickness um
ILM - RPE	683	13.4	373

Comments	Physician's Signature	SW Ver: 3.0.0.64
High-definition mode		Copyright 2008 Carl Zeiss Meditec, Inc. All Rights Reserved Page 1 of 1

4. What is the diagnosis?

5. What are the risk factors?

6. What is the treatment?

7. What are the complications of surgery?

8. What is the prognosis after surgery?

4. ERM with cystoid macular edema.

5. Although most epiretinal membranes are idiopathic and occur in women > 50 years of age, risk factors include prior intraocular surgery, intraocular inflammation, retinal vascular occlusion, sickle cell retinopathy, telangiectasia, diabetic retinopathy, arteriole macroaneurysm, previous vitreous hemorrhage, trauma, macular holes, intraocular tumors such as angiomas and hamartomas, telangiectasis, retinal arteriolar macroaneurysms, inherited retinal dystrophies such as retinitis pigmentosa, previous laser photocoagulation, and previous cryotherapy.

6. An ERM rarely requires treatment. Pars plana vitrectomy and membrane peel are considered in patients with reduced acuity (<20/40) or who are symptomatic.

7. The most common complication is cataracts (nuclear sclerosis; posterior subcapsular is due to lens touch or the use of intraocular gas). Retinal tears occur in up to 5% of cases. The most common late complication is RRD (probably as a result of contraction of the vitreous into the sclerotomy sites). Rare complications include phototoxicity (especially when intraocular dyes such as ICG are used), endophthalmitis, and visual field defects.

8. About 80%–90% of patients have an improvement in visual acuity of ≥ 2 Snellen lines. Recurrent ERM occurs in up to 5% of patients.

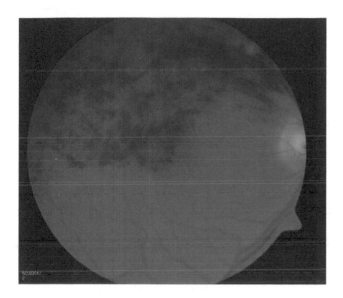

A 65-year-old man presents with a sudden, painless, quadrantic visual field defect.

1. What does the fundus photo show?
2. What is the differential diagnosis?
3. What test would you obtain?

Additional information: the FA shows:

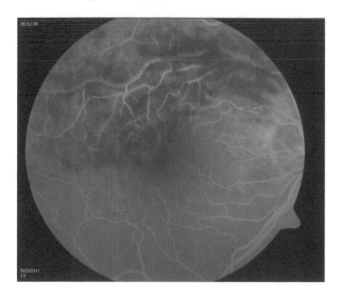

4. How do you interpret this test?
5. What is the diagnosis?

1. Dilated, tortuous, superior retinal vein with superficial, retinal hemorrhages, and cotton-wool spots in a wedge-shaped area radiating from an arteriovenous crossing.

2. BRVO, venous stasis retinopathy, ocular ischemic syndrome, hypertensive retinopathy, leukemic retinopathy, retinopathy of anemia, diabetic retinopathy, papilledema, papillophlebitis (in young patients).

3. FA; consider a wide-field FA to evaluate for peripheral ischemia. OCT is often also performed to evaluate for amount and location of macular edema. OCTA shows the ischemic areas and can delineate neovascularization.

4. The FA shows delayed retinal venous filling in the superior branch of the central retinal vein, blocked fluorescence from retinal hemorrhages, and capillary nonperfusion in the area supplied by the involved retinal vein.

5. BRVO.

6. What are the risk factors for this disease?

7. What are the different forms?

8. How would you work up this patient?

9. What is the treatment?

10. What is the prognosis?

6. BRVO is associated with hypertension (50%–70% of cases), coronary artery disease, diabetes mellitus, and peripheral vascular disease. Rare associations include: hypercoagulable states (eg, macroglobulinemia, cryoglobulinemia), hyperviscosity states (polycythemia vera, Waldenström macroglobulinemia), SLE, syphilis, sarcoid, homocystinuria, malignancies (eg, multiple myeloma, polycythemia vera, leukemia), optic nerve drusen, and external compression. In younger patients, associated with oral contraceptive pills, collagen vascular disease, acquired immunodeficiency syndrome (AIDS), protein S/protein C/antithrombin III deficiency, factor XII (Hageman factor) deficiency, antiphospholipid antibody syndrome, or activated protein C resistance (factor V Leiden PCR assay).

7. There are 2 types of BRVO: nonischemic (64%; defined as < 5 disc areas of capillary nonperfusion on FA) and ischemic (defined as ≥ 5 disc areas of capillary nonperfusion on FA).

8. In older patients, obtain fasting blood glucose, glycosylated hemoglobin and blood pressure measurement to rule out hypertension and diabetes. Consider checking: CBC with differential, platelets, PT/PTT, ANA, (RF), ACE, ESR, serum protein electrophoresis, lipid profile, hemoglobin electrophoresis (in African Americans), sedimentation rate, Venereal Disease Research Laboratory (VDRL or RPR, FTA-ABS or MHA-TP depending on the clinical situation.

   In younger patients (<40 years old) and in whom a hypercoagulable state is being considered, check HIV status, functional protein S assay, functional protein C assay, functional antithrombin III assay (type II heparin-binding mutation), antiphospholipid antibody titer, lupus anticoagulant, anticardiolipin antibody titer (IgG and IgM), homocysteine level (if elevated, test for folate, B12, and creatinine), factor XII (Hageman factor) levels, and activated protein C resistance (factor V Leiden mutation PCR assay). If these tests are normal and clinical suspicion for a hypercoagulable state still exists, then order: plasminogen antigen assay, heparin cofactor II assay, thrombin time, reptilase time, and fibrinogen functional assay.

9. *Anti-VEGF:* the BRAVO study reported better results than laser using monthly intravitreal injection of ranibizumab (Lucentis) for macular edema. Bevacizumab is used off-label for macular edema. The VIBRANT study reported better results than laser using monthly intravitreal injection of aflibercept (Eylea) for six injections, then every other month. Anti-VEGF is the first-line therapy. If vision is good, the practitioner can observe to see if spontaneous resolution occurs.

   Laser: the BVOS reported that macular grid/focal photocoagulation should be performed when macular edema lasts > 3 months and vision is < 20/40. If rubeosis, disc/retinal neovascularization, or neovascular glaucoma develops, then quadrantic scatter laser photocoagulation to the area of ischemia. Prophylactic laser was not evaluated in the BVOS and is not recommended.

   Steroids: the GENEVA (Global Evaluation of Implantable Dexamethasone in Retinal Vein Occlusion with Macular Edema) study reported positive results using an intravitreal injection of a sustained-release intravitreal dexamethasone implant (Ozurdex) for macular edema.

10. Thirty percent have spontaneous recovery and > 50% maintain vision > 20/40 after 1 year. Ten percent have BRVO in the fellow eye.

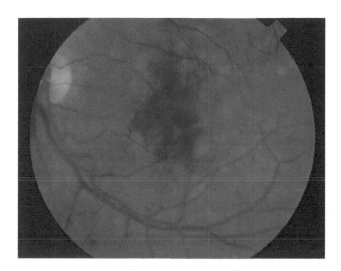

A 22-year-old woman reports decreased vision with photopsias.

1. What does the fundus photo show?
2. What is the differential diagnosis?
3. What test would you obtain?

Additional information: the FA shows:

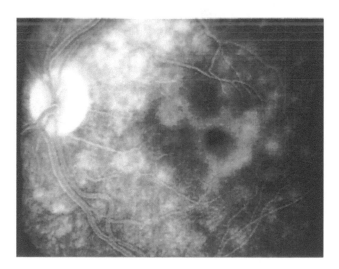

4. How do you interpret this test?
5. What is the diagnosis?
6. What are the risk factors for this disease?
7. What is the treatment?
8. What is the prognosis?

1. Multifocal, deep gray-white retinal lesions with orange yellow granularity of the fovea.

2. White dot syndrome including MEWDS, APMPPE, MCP, PIC, and birdshot chorioretinopathy.

3. FA (see below), FAF shows hyper-autofluorescent areas corresponding to lesions. OCT shows discontinuities in the outer retina (outer segment ellipsoid zone and external limiting membrane) corresponding to the lesions. Enlarged blind spot and central or paracentral scotoma on visual field testing. ICG show hyperfluorescent lesions that outnumber fundus lesions.

4. The FA demonstrates early punctate hyperfluorescence in a wreath-like pattern with late staining that correspond to the lesions.

5. MEWDS.

6. Healthy young woman aged 10–50 years old; may be associated with prodromal viral illness.

7. No treatment needed; self-limited disease.

8. Good, but up to 10% can have recurrences.

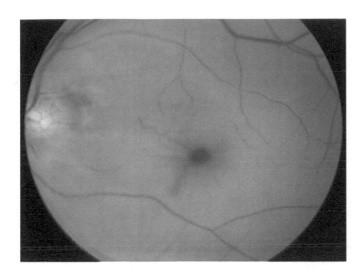

A 75-year-old woman presents with sudden, painless, loss of vision.

1. What does the fundus photo show?
2. What is the differential diagnosis?
3. What testing may be helpful?

Additional information: if the FA shows:

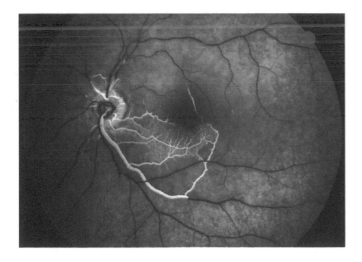

4. What is the diagnosis?
5. What are the risk factors for this disease?
6. How would you work up this patient?
7. What is the treatment?
8. What is the prognosis?

1. Cherry red spot.

2. The differential diagnosis of a cherry red spot is mainly central retinal artery occlusion and metabolic storage diseases such as Hurler disease, Tay–Sachs disease (GM2 gangliosidosis), mucopolysaccharidosis type VII (MPS VII, Sly syndrome), Farber disease, GM1 gangliosidoses, Niemann Pick disease, Sandhoff disease, Shprintzen–Goldberg syndrome, Hallervorden–Spatz disease, Krabbe disease, metachromatic leukodystrophy; also trauma (commotio retinae), ophthalmic artery occlusion (cherry red spot may be present but usually is not), and toxicity from methanol, quinine, dapsone, and carbon monoxide,

3. FA shows delayed filling of retinal arteries and delayed arteriovenous transit time. OCT in acute shows increased reflectivity and thickening of the inner retina, and decreased reflectivity of the outer retina. Late OCT shows retina thinning. OCTA shows the areas of nonperfusion.

4. CRAO with patent cilioretinal artery.

5. Atherosclerosis, cardiac valvular disease, hypercoagulable states including oral contraceptive use, and collagen vascular diseases.

6. Carotid Doppler ultrasound and cardiac echocardiography. In older patients, obtain ESR and C-reactive protein to rule out giant cell arteritis. If workup is negative, then consider laboratory tests for hypercoagulable state depending on the clinical situation. Some have suggested that an emergent vascular medicine workup should be performed.

7. There is no effective treatment. Any chance of success to limit visual loss must be instituted within 90 minutes of onset making intervention unlikely. All attempts at treatment are based on the idea of moving the embolus (ie, lowering IOP rapidly with anterior chamber paracentesis, systemic acetazolamide, digital ocular massage, topical ocular hypotensive drops, carbogen treatment), and should be performed before imaging tests to prevent vision loss.

8. Poor prognosis. In the presence of cilioretinal artery sparing-CRAO, visual prognosis is better with 80% having ≥ 20/50 vision. Neovascular complications can occur in 15%–20% of patients.

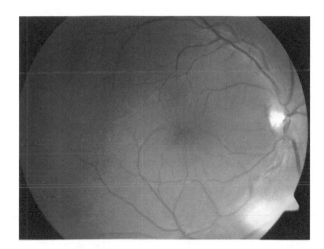

A 62-year-old woman complains of gradual decreased vision OD. Her BSCVA is 20/50 with a mild hyperopic shift.

1. What does the fundus photo show?

2. What is the diagnosis and differential diagnosis?

3. What are the possible etiologies?

4. What tests would you obtain?

Additional information: the patient underwent uncomplicated cataract surgery 3 months ago. The FA shows:

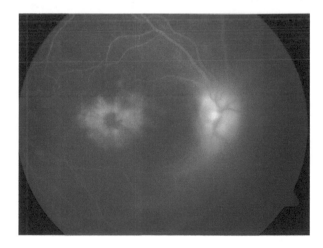

5. What does the FA demonstrate?

6. What is the diagnosis?

7. What are the risk factors for this disease?

8. What is the treatment?

1. Decreased foveal reflex with intraretinal cystic changes.

2. CME. The differential diagnosis of CME is pseudocystoid macular edema (no leakage on FA; X-linked retinoschisis, Goldmann–Favre syndrome, and nicotinic acid maculopathy), macular hole (stage 1), pseudohole, foveal retinoschisis, central serous chorioretinopathy, and choroidal neovascular membrane.

3. The etiology of CME can be remembered with the mnemonic **DEPRIVEN**: Diabetes, Epinephrine, Pars planitis, RP, Irvine–Gass syndrome, Venous occlusion, E_2 prostaglandin, Nicotinic acid maculopathy (does not leak). However, this is not a complete list, and other causes include uveitis, macular or retinal telangiectasia, retinal vasculitis, epiretinal membrane, hereditary retinal dystrophies (dominant CME as well as RP), hypertensive retinopathy, radiation retinopathy, exudative AMD, occult RRD, intraocular tumors, collagen vascular diseases, hypotony, and chronic inflammation.

4. FA (see below), OCT shows the typical cystoid spaces with loss of the normal foveal contour and increased retinal thickening; may also show subretinal fluid.

5. Leakage from perifoveal capillaries with petalloid appearance.

6. Pseudophakic CME (Irvine–Gass syndrome).

7. Clinical CME is rare after uncomplicated small incision phacoemulsification cataract extraction occurring in 2%–5% of cases; however, angiographic- or OCT-based CME is seen in 15%–30% of cases. In complicated cases, reports as high as 60%. Risk factors include diabetic retinopathy, uveitis, glaucoma (especially with prostaglandin analog therapy), retinal vein occlusion, and preexisting epiretinal membrane.

8. Topical NSAID drops are usually tried first (a meta-analysis of four randomized clinical trials showed a benefit). A combination of steroid and NSAID drops are added in more resistant cases. Periocular and intravitreal steroids, and anti-VEGF injections have been used in difficult cases.

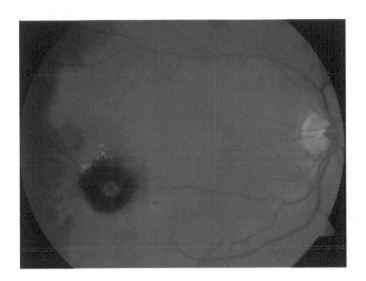

A 72-year-old woman is found to have a fundus abnormality on routine examination.

1. What does the fundus photo show?
2. What is the differential diagnosis?
3. What test would you obtain?

Additional information: the FA shows:

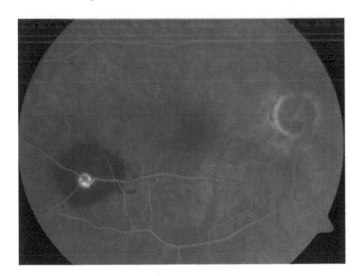

4. What is the diagnosis?
5. What are the risk factor(s) for this disease?
6. What is the treatment?

1. Lipid exudates and hemorrhage surrounding a focal dilation of a retinal artery.

2. Retinal artery macroaneurysm, Coats disease, von Hippel–Lindau, branch retinal vein occlusion, diabetic retinopathy, radiation retinopathy.

3. FA, if too much blood then ICG angiogram should be performed.

4. Retinal artery macroaneurysm.

5. Strong association with hypertension.

6. Usually none required; often spontaneously regress after bleed. Anti-VEGF agents have been tried with success when macular edema occurs in association with the macroaneurysm. In the past, laser treatment adjacent to the macroaneurysm has been reported, but is controversial. In severe bleeding, surgery has been advocated especially with submacular hemorrhage or nonclearing vitreous hemorrhage.

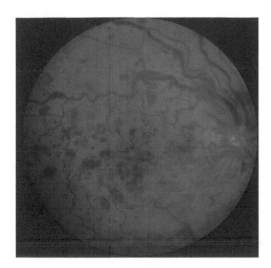

A 73-year-old man presents with painless, sudden decrease in vision that he noticed upon awakening.

1. What does the fundus photo show?
2. What is the differential diagnosis?
3. What testing would you obtain?

Additional information: the FA shows:

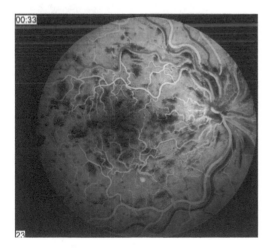

4. What does the FA show, and what is the diagnosis?
5. What are the risk factors for this disease?
6. What are the different forms?

1. Disc edema with tortuous, dilated retinal veins and intraretinal hemorrhages in all four quadrants.

2. CRVO, hemiretinal vein occlusion, BRVO, ocular ischemic syndrome, radiation retinopathy, retinal artery occlusion, ARN.

3. FA to evaluate arteriovenous transit time and nonperfusion; wide angle FA is helpful to evaluate the extent of nonperfusion. OCT to evaluate for macular edema.

4. The FA shows no filling of the central retinal vein and blocking from hemorrhages, which is characteristic of a CRVO.

5. Risk factors for CRVO include age (90% of cases > 50 years old), hypertension (up to 75% of cases), diabetes mellitus (up to 10% of cases), hyperlipidemia, elevated IOP/glaucoma, use of oral contraceptive pill, smoking. Less common predispositions are hypercoagulable states including: polycythemia, multiple myeloma, Waldenström macroglobulinemia, hyperhomocysteinemia, lupus anticoagulant and antiphospholipid antibodies, dysfibrinogenemia, activated protein C resistance (factor V Leiden mutation), protein C deficiency, protein S deficiency, antithrombin deficiency, prothrombin gene mutation, factor Xll deficiency.

6. Impending CRVO is when a patient is asymptomatic or complains of episodic episodes of blurry vision with venous dilation, retinal hemorrhages, and delayed circulation time. Nonischemic CRVO usually has vision > 20/200 and minimal capillary nonperfusion. It is the most common form (75%). Ischemic CRVO often has poor vision (< 20/200), severe ERG changes, marked relative afferent pupillary defect (RAPD), and significant retinal ischemia (≥10 disk areas of capillary nonperfusion on FA). Patient is more likely to develop ischemic complications. Ten percent of nonischemic patients (absent or mild RAPD) will become ischemic.

7. What laboratory evaluation should be performed?
8. What is the treatment?
9. What is the prognosis?

7. In older patients, obtain fasting blood glucose, glycosylated hemoglobin and blood pressure measurement to rule out hypertension and diabetes. Consider checking: CBC with differential, platelets, PT/PTT, ANA, RF, ESR, serum protein electrophoresis, lipid profile, hemoglobin electrophoresis (in African American) depending on the clinical situation. In younger patients (<40 years old) and in whom a hypercoagulable state is being considered, check: HIV status, functional protein S assay, functional protein C assay, functional antithrombin III assay (type II heparin-binding mutation), antiphospholipid antibody titer, lupus anticoagulant, anticardiolipin antibody titer (IgG and IgM), homocysteine level (if elevated, test for do not spell out folate, B12, and creatinine), factor XII (Hageman factor) levels, and activated protein C resistance (factor V Leiden mutation PCR assay). If these tests are normal and clinical suspicion for a hypercoagulable state still exists, then order: plasminogen antigen assay, heparin cofactor II assay, thrombin time, reptilase time, and fibrinogen functional assay.

8. *Anti-VEGF:* intravitreal injections of ranibizumab (Lucentis; CRUISE Study), aflibercept (Eylea; COPERNICUS and GALILEO studies), and off-label bevacizumab (Avastin) have been shown to be beneficial.

   Steroids: intravitreal steroid injections were beneficial in the SCORE and SCORE2 studies. The dexamethasone implant (Ozurdex) has also been shown to be beneficial in the GENEVA study. The fluocinolone acetonide implant (Iluvien) was shown to be beneficial in the FAVOR study. Usually second-line therapy to anti-VEGF agents due to cataract and elevated IOP.

   Laser: has not been shown to be beneficial in macular edema due to CRVO; however, panretinal photocoagulation when neovascular complications occur is proven (CVOS conclusion). Early treatment with PRP is not proven.

9. Younger patients (<50 years old) have better prognosis. In nonischemic cases, prognosis is good with improvement in vision in almost 50%. Final vision is related to baseline vision: those > 20/60 usually do well; those < 20/200 do not. Follow patients frequently in first 6–8 months to evaluate for ischemic complications and treat any macular edema. Conversion to ischemic occurs in 15% of cases within 4–6 months, and 30% in 3 years. Risk factors for ischemic complications: (1) Extent of nonperfusion, (2) large amounts of retinal hemorrhages, (3) short duration of CRVO, and (4) male sex.

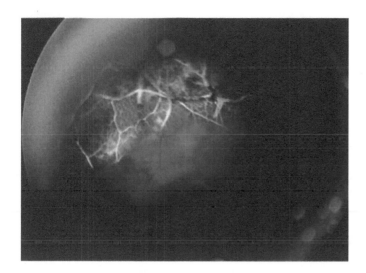

A 32-year-old man presents for a routine exam. He has no past ocular history or visual complaints.

1. What does the fundus photo show?
2. What is the differential diagnosis?
3. What is the diagnosis?
4. What is the prognosis and management?

1. Branching white lines with surrounding hyperpigmentation in the retinal periphery.

2. Lattice degeneration, atrophic retinal holes, cobblestone degeneration, retinoschisis, chorioretinal scar, CHRPE, bear tracks, vitreoretinal traction.

3. Lattice degeneration.

4. Perform a careful dilated fundus examination with scleral depression to rule out retinal tears, holes, or other pathology. In the absence of symptoms, the patient is followed with observation. Lattice occurs in approximately 10% of the general population, and prophylactic treatment is not recommended. When associated with symptoms and other retinal pathology, consider laser retinopexy or cryotherapy depending on the clinical situation.

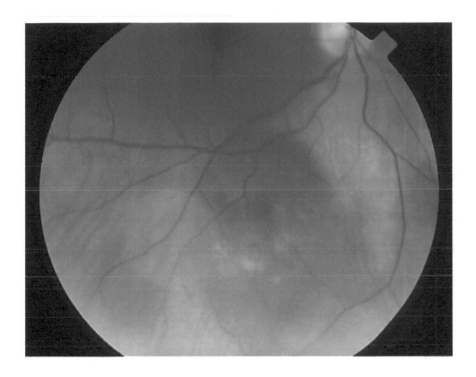

A 58-year-old woman is noted to have a retinal abnormality.

1. What does the photo show?
2. What is the diagnosis?
3. What associated findings can occur?
4. What are the risks for malignant transformation?
5. How would you manage this patient?

1. Flat, pigmented lesion with drusen.

2. Choroidal nevus.

3. Overlying drusen and hypopigmented ring/halo around the base. Multiple nevi are associated with neurofibromatosis.

4. Risk of transformation is 4%. Presence of a risk factor increases relative risk ~3 ×. Risk factors can be remembered with the mnemonics:

   TFSOM-DIM (to find small ocular melanoma doing imaging): **T**hickness (>2 mm), **F**luid (subretinal), **S**ymptoms (visual, usually flashes or floaters), **O**range pigment (lipofuscin), **M**elanoma hollow on ultrasound, **DIa**Meter (>5 mm on fundus photography)

   MOLES: **M**ushroom shape, **O**range pigment, **L**arge size (>2 mm thickness, >5 mm diameter), **E**nlarging tumor, **S**ubretinal fluid

5. Serial fundus photography to document size and examine on an annual basis to monitor for growth or change in appearance. Thickening is assessed with B-scan ultrasonography and OCT. Evaluate more frequently if changes occur.

Index of Cases

Index